Electroanatomical
Mapping

Electroanatomical Mapping: An Atlas for Clinicians

EDITED BY

Amin Al-Ahmad, MD

Cardiac Arrhythmia Service
Stanford University Medical Center
Stanford, CA
USA

David Callans, MD

Cardiology Division
Hospital of University of Pennsylvania
Philadelphia, PA
USA

Henry Hsia, MD

Cardiac Arrhythmia Service
Stanford University Medical Center
Stanford, CA
USA

Andrea Natale, MD

Cardiac Arrhythmia Service
Stanford University Medical Center
Stanford, CA
USA

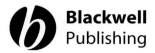
Blackwell
Publishing

Blackwell Publishing, Inc., 350 Main Street, Malden, Massachusetts 02148-5020, USA
Blackwell Publishing Ltd, 9600 Garsington Road, Oxford OX4 2DQ, UK
Blackwell Science Asia Pty Ltd, 550 Swanston Street, Carlton, Victoria 3053, Australia

First published 2008

1   2008

ISBN: 978-1-4051-5702-5

Library of Congress Cataloging-in-Publication Data

Electroanatomical mapping : an atlas for clinicians / edited by Amin Al-Ahmad ... [et al.].
    p. ; cm.
Includes bibliographical references and index.
    ISBN 978-1-4051-5702-5 (alk. paper)
    1. Arrhythmia–Imaging–Atlases. 2. Catheter ablation–Atlases. 3. Electrocardiography–
Atlases. I. Al-Ahmad, Amin.
    [DNLM: 1. Arrhythmia–diagnosis–Atlases. 2. Arrhythmia–surgery–Atlases. 3. Catheter
Ablation–methods–Atlases. 4. Electrophysiologic Techniques, Cardiac–methods–Atlases.
    5. Image Processing, Computer-Assisted–methods–Atlases. WG 17 E38 2008]

RC685.A65E435 2008

616.1'28–dc22

                                                                                2007031203

A catalogue record for this title is available from the British Library

Commissioning Editor: Gina Almond
Development Editor: Fiona Pattison
Editorial Assistant: Victoria Pitman
Production Controller: Debbie Wyer

Set in 9.5pt/12pt Minion by Newgen Imaging Systems (P) Ltd, Chennai, India
Printed and bound in Singapore by Markono Print Media Pte Ltd

For further information on Blackwell Publishing, visit our website:
www.blackwellcardiology.com

Contents

Contributors

Amin Al-Ahmad, MD
Cardiac Electrophysiology and Arrhythmia Service
Stanford University Medical Center
Stanford, CA, USA

Moataz Aly, MD
Assistant Lecturer
Critical Care Department
Cairo University, Cairo, Egypt
and
Research Fellow
Section of Cardiac Electrophysiology and Pacing
Department of Cardiovascular Medicine
Cleveland Clinic
Cleveland, OH, USA

James David Allred, MD
Cardiac Electrophysiology
Division of Cardiovascular Disease
University of Alabama at Birmingham
Birmingham, AL, USA

Daejoon Anh, MD
Cardiac Electrophysiology Fellow
Stanford University
Stanford, CA, USA

Rupa Bala, MD
The Electrophysiology Service
Cardiovascular Division
University of Pennsylvania Health System
Philadelphia, PA, USA

David J. Callans, MD, FACC, FHRS
The Electrophysiology Service, Cardiovascular Division
University of Pennsylvania Health System
Philadelphia, PA, USA

Riccardo Cappato, MD
Director
Center of Clinical Arrhythmia and Electrophysiology
IRCCS Policlinico San Donato
San Donato Milanese
Milan, Italy

William M. Castell, BS, RCIS
Testamur NASPExAM AP/EP
San Francisco, CA, USA

Henry A. Chen, MD
Cardiac Electrophysiology and Arrhythmia Service
Stanford University Medical Center
Stanford, CA, USA

Luigi Di Biase, MD
Research Fellow
Department of Cardiovascular Medicine
Section of Cardiac Electrophysiology and Pacing
Cleveland Clinic Cleveland,
OH, USA
and
University of Foggia
Foggia, Italy

Harish Doppalapudi, MD
Assistant Professor of Medicine
Division of Cardiovascular Disease
University of Alabama at Birmingham
Birmingham, AL, USA

N. A. Mark Estes III, MD
Professor of Medicine
Tufts University School of Medicine
Director, New England Cardiac Arrhythmia Center
Tufts-New England Medical Center
Boston, MA, USA

Tamer Fahmy, MD, PHD
Cardiac Electrophysiology and Critical Care Medicine
Critical Care Medicine Department
Cairo University Hospitals
CAI, Egypt

Gregory K. Feld, MD
Professor of Medicine
Director, Cardiac Electrophysiology Program
University of California San Diego Medical Center
San Diego,
CA, USA

Blair Halperin, MD
Heart Rhythm Center
Providence St. Vincent Hospital
Portland, OR, USA

Richard Hongo, MD
Cardiac Electrophysiology
Marin General Hospital
San Francisco, CA, USA

Henry H. Hsia, MD
Cardiac Electrophysiology and Arrhythmia Service
Stanford University Medical Center
Stanford, CA, USA

Jeff Hsing, MD, MS
Division of Cardiovascular Medicine
Stanford University Medical Center
Stanford, CA, USA

Linda L. Huffer, MD
Walter Reed Army Medical Center
Washington, DC, USA

Warren M. Jackman, MD
George Lynn Cross Research Professor
Co-Director, Cardiac Arrhythmia Research Institute
University of Oklahoma Health Sciences Center
Oklahoma City, OK, USA

Jason T. Jacobson, MD
Assistant Professor
Division of Cardiology
Department of Medicine at Northwestern University
Feinberg School of Medicine
Chicago, IL, USA

G. Neal Kay, MD
Professor of Medicine
Director, Clinical Cardiac Electrophysiology
University of Alabama at Birmingham
Birmingham, AL, USA

Yung R. Lau, MD
Division of Pediatric Cardiology
University of Alabama at Birmingham
Birmingham, AL, USA

Kevin J. Makati, MD
Fellow, Cardiac Electrophysiology
Department of Cardiovascular Medicine
Tufts University-New England Medical Center
Clinical Associate
Department of Medicine
Tufts University School of Medicine
Boston, MA, USA

Sumeet K. Mainigi, MD
Associate Director of Electrophysiology
Albert Einstein Medical Center
Philadelphia,
PA, USA

Pirooz Mofrad, MD
Cardiac Electrophysiology and Arrhythmia Service
Stanford University Medical Center
Stanford, CA, USA

Hiroshi Nakagawa, MD, PHD
Professor of Medicine
Cardiac Arrhythmia Research Institute
University of Oklahoma Health Sciences Centre
Oklahoma City, OK, USA

Andrea Natale, MD, FACC, FHRS
Department of Cardiology
Stanford University
Palo Alto, CA, USA

Dimpi Patel, DO
Electrophysiology Research Fellow
Section of Cardiac Electrophysiology and Pacing
Department of Cardiovascular Medicine
Cleveland Clinic
Cleveland,
OH, USA

Luis C. Saenz Morales, MD
Cardiologist-Electrophysiologist
Head of the Electrophysiology Service
Fundacion Cardio Infantil-Instituto de Cardiologia
Bogota, Colombia

Robert A. Schweikert, MD
Director, EP Clinical Operations
Section of Cardiac Electrophysiology and Pacing
Department of Cardiovascular Medicine
Cleveland Clinic
Cleveland, OH, USA

William Stevenson, MD
Professor of Medicine
Harvard Medical School
Director, Clinical Cardiac Electrophysiology Program
Brigham and Women's Hospital
Boston, MA, USA

Jonathan S. Sussman, MD
Cardiac Electrophysiology
Gagnon Heart Hospital
Morristown Memorial Hospital
Morristown,
NJ, USA

Craig A. Swygman
Senior Electrophysiology Technologist
Heart Rhythm Center
Providence St. Vincent Hospital
Portland, Oregon, USA

John Triedman, MD
Associate Professor of Pediatrics
Department of Cardiology
Children's Hospital Boston
Harvard University
Boston, MA, USA

Miguel Vacca, MD, MSC
Cardiologist Electrophysiologist
Master in Clinical Epidemiology and Research
Arrhythmia Service
Fundación Cardioinfantil, Instituto de Cardiología
Bogotá, Colombia

George F. Van Hare, MD
Professor of Pediatrics
Lucile Packard Children's Hospital
Stanford University
Palo Alto, CA, USA

Paul J. Wang, MD
Professor of Medicine
Stanford University School of Medicine
Stanford,
CA, USA

Oussama M.Wazni, MD
Cardiac Pacing and Electrophysiology
Director, Clinical Atrial Fibrillation Research
Associate Director, Cleveland Clinic Cardiovascular
Coordinating Center for Research
Cleveland Clinic
Cleveland,
OH, USA

Takumi Yamada, MD, PHD
Cardiac Electrophysiology
Division of Cardiovascular Disease
University of Alabama at Birmingham
Birmingham, AL, USA

Paul C. Zei, MD
Cardiac Electrophysiology and Arrhythmia Service
Stanford University Medical Center
Stanford, CA, USA

Foreword

For decades electrophysiologists faced the challenge of assimilating information from the surface ECG, intracardiac multielectrode recordings, and fluoroscopic images to localize the source of an arrhythmia, elucidate the path of an arrhythmia circuit, and characterize the electrophysiolgic (EP) substrate. Those who were the most experienced were the most cautious in attempting to extrapolate the detail afforded by limited recording and display capabilities. The last decade has seen the much-needed evolution of three-dimensional electroanatomic mapping systems and intracardiac imaging tools. These 3-D mapping systems facilitate the display of electrical activation and local bipolar or unipolar voltage characteristics. These systems have revolutionized electrophysiology and permit online color-coded computerized display of electrical information used as targets for successful catheter-based ablation procedures. An increased understanding and appreciation of the importance of anatomy to the electrophysiologist has occurred and anatomic targets are now an integral part of many ablation strategies.

The publication of this important color atlas of EP cases that incorporates detailed images from 3-D cardiac mapping systems and other imaging tools such as intracardiac echo is timed with their general acceptance as integral to the success of most ablation procedures. Each of the co-editors of the text has made seminal contributions to the field and has now combined their efforts to provide the readership with an invaluable source book. Through the contribution of cases from leaders in the EP field, the editors have provided us an organized and highly readable "how to" text on the utilization of these exciting imaging and recording tools for localizing and ablating arrhythmias. For each case the elctroanatomic mapping information is correlated with clinical, surface ECG, and electrogram data. This book will certainly be enjoyed by all in electrophysiology who are dedicated to marrying advances in technology with the fundamentals of electrophysiology. Whether novice or expert, the appeal and educational value of this case-based-approach instruction technique are guaranteed to the reader.

Dr. Francis Marchlinski
University of Pennsylvania, USA
August 2007

CHAPTER 1

Electroanatomical mapping technologies

Jeff Hsing, MD, *Paul J. Wang,* MD, *& Amin Al-Ahmad,* MD

Introduction

Mapping of cardiac arrhythmias is the process of identifying, characterizing, and localizing an arrhythmia. Mapping forms the foundation for guiding ablation therapies and directing intervention. The principles and techniques for mapping have advanced considerably over the past decades. With improved understanding of cardiac arrhythmias including anatomical and structural relationships, the concept of combining the electrical information obtained using mapping catheters to anatomical information guided by catheter position and contact has been crucial in the understanding and success of catheter ablation.

The principle behind electroanatomical mapping involves using mapping catheters that collect electrical information from the tip of the catheter, such as the timing of the electrogram with respect to a stable timing reference as well as the local voltage, and combining this with catheter tip location information, where the electrical information was obtained. In this fashion, a three-dimensional surface geometry that represents the chamber of interest is created. The surface anatomical geometry can be color coded to represent timing or voltage. This allows the operator to examine an activation map of the arrhythmia wave front. In addition, the operator may be able to visualize areas of scar or areas of interest such as fractionated electrograms or anatomical landmarks.

Electroanatomical Mapping, 1st edition. Edited by A. Al-Ahmad, D. Callans, H. Hsia and A. Natale.
© 2008 Blackwell Publishing, ISBN: 9781405157025.

Current electroanatomical mapping systems utilize either contact or noncontact mapping. Contact mapping relies on the mapping catheter making contact with the endocardial border and sequentially acquiring location data points over many cardiac cycles. Current systems that use this technique include CARTO™, NavX™, and Realtime Position Management. Noncontact mapping is based on a concept of simultaneously acquiring electrogram data of an entire chamber without making physical contact with the endocardial border. The only system that currently uses this technique is the EnSite Array™.

Three-dimensional mapping systems are currently being utilized by the majority of cardiac electrophysiology laboratories in the United States as well as internationally for mapping and ablating a variety of arrhythmias.

Electroanatomical mapping systems

The Biosense CARTO™ system

The first description of the use of nonfluoroscopic electroanatomical mapping *in vivo* by Ben-Haim *et al.* in 1996 heralded the beginning of the use of this technology for catheter ablation [1]. The technology, which became Biosense CARTO™, was the first three-dimensional electroanatomical system. In the initial study, CARTO™ was used to map and navigate the right atrium during both normal sinus rhythm and atrial flutter, proving that nonfluoroscopic electroanatomical mapping techniques were feasible *in vivo*. The Biosense CARTO™ system has been extensively validated and has been used to map a variety of arrhythmias in all cardiac chambers.

The technology can be used for mapping ventricular tachycardias, atrial tachycardias, and identification of scar using voltage map [2–6].

The Biosense CARTO™ system utilizes a magnetic field sensor incorporated in the tip of a deflectable quadripolar mapping catheter (NAVISTAR™) and an external magnetic field emitter located under the patient and the operating table. The external magnetic field emitter utilizes three coils that generate an ultra-low magnetic field (between 5×10^{-6} and 5×10^{-5} T) that codes the mapping space around the patient's chest with both temporal and spatial information [7]. Spatial information is encoded in the decaying magnetic field as a function of distance from the coil. The magnetic field sensor at the tip of the catheter measures the strength of the magnetic field from each coil, this can then be used to calculate the distance from each coil. The location of the catheter in space is computed as the intersection of the distance from the three coils (Figure 1.1). The magnetic field contains the information needed to determine the sensor location in six degrees of freedom, dimensions (x, y, z), and orientation (roll, yaw, pitch).

An electroanatomical map is generated when the mapping catheter is manipulated around the cardiac chamber and data points are sequentially collected. Data collection includes three-dimensional spatial location corresponding to electrical data of local activation time relative to the reference location. By sequentially acquiring data from multiple endocardial points, a detailed three-dimensional electroanatomical map is generated. As more points are acquired, the more detailed the map is.

To correct for minor patient movement, a reference is used, which is located on the patient's back (REF-STAR with QuikPatch). The mapping system subtracts the location of the mapping catheter from the simultaneous location of the reference patch to compensate for any patient motion.

Recently, Biosense CARTO™ has introduced a module that allows for the incorporation of a pre-acquired three-dimensional image obtained using computer tomography (CT) or magnetic resonance imaging (MRI) into the electroanatomical map as a fully registered image. This new software, CARTOMERGE™, merges the CT and MRI data with the electroanatomical map obtained

during the procedure (Figure 1.2). This technology is useful for the ablation of atrial fibrillation, where the ablation strategy may often be anatomical and an understanding of each patient's individual variation may be useful [8–10]. Recently, Fahmy *et al.* showed that posterior wall landmarks at the pulmonary vein and left atrium junction are the most accurate landmarks for image registration and integration of cardiac CT data with CARTO™ [11].

Potential limitations to the Biosense CARTO™ system are the sequential mapping on a point-by-point and beat-by-beat basis. This limits the use of this technology for unsustained or unstable rhythms as they are difficult or time consuming to map. Despite this limitation, for some unstable arrhythmias, difficult-to-induce rhythms, or sustain rhythms, generating a voltage map in normal

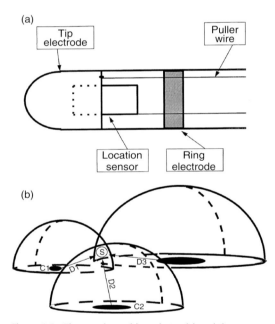

Figure 1.1 The new locatable catheter (a) and the process of location determination (b). (a) The locatable catheter is composed of tip and ring electrodes and a location sensor totally embedded within the catheter. (b) Process of location determination. A location pad is composed of three coils (C1, C2, C3) that generate a magnetic field that decays as a function of distance from that coil. The sensor (S) measures the strength of the field, and the distance from each coil (D1, D2, D3) can be measured. The location of the sensor is determined from the intersection of the theoretical spheres whose radii are the distances measured by the sensor. (Reprinted with permission from Reference 7.)

sinus rhythm may help the operator gain insight on potential arrhythmia circuits in the case of and may result in a successful ablation outcome. Another potential limitation includes the possibility that the system accuracy may be compromised by the presence of any material that may disrupt the magnetic field. As the spatial orientation is calculated from the measured strength of the generated magnetic fields from the coils, any disturbance to the magnetic field or strength may lead to inaccurate distance measurements, although this would be rare in a well-shielded modern electrophysiology laboratory. Additionally, the Biosense CARTO™ system is

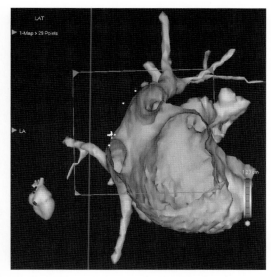

Figure 1.2 Registered three-dimensional left atrial surface reconstruction showing the left pulmonary veins during pulmonary vein isolation for atrial fibrillation using CARTOMERGE™.

sensitive to patient motion because of the location of the coils underneath the patient. This necessitates remapping of the arrhythmia if significant patient movement is detected and can be time consuming or lead to inaccuracies if not detected relatively quickly. In addition, significant movement of the internal reference catheter can also lead to map inaccuracies. Finally, the Biosense CARTO™ system requires the use of proprietary single-use catheters made by Biosense Webster and does not support the use of other manufacturer catheters.

St. Jude Medical EnSite Array™ system

In 1998, a second mapping system, EnSite 3000, later renamed EnSite Array, by St. Jude Medical (St. Paul, MN) was described by Schilling *et al.* They compared the left ventricular electroanatomical map of the new noncontact mapping system against a traditional contact map of 13 patients undergoing left ventricular ablation [12]. The EnSite Array™ system is a noncontact mapping system that allows for simultaneous recordings from multiple sites within a single cardiac chamber. In addition to the ability of the system to map sustained atrial or ventricular arrhythmias, the system can be used for mapping of nonsustained or hemodynamically unstable arrhythmias. It can also be used to map multiple cardiac cycles allowing the ability to visualize changes in the electrical map over time. The system can be used in conjunction with the EnSite NavX™ system.

The system utilizes a 9-Fr catheter with a 7.6 mL (18 × 40 mm) ellipsoid balloon surrounded by 64 multielectrode array (MEA) [12] (Figure 1.3). Each of the 64 electrodes is electrically insulated and has a 0.025-in. break in the insulation,

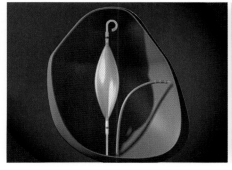
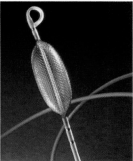

Figure 1.3 EnSite Array™ noncontact system with MEA. (Courtesy of St. Jude Medical.)

allowing it to function as unipolar electrodes. Raw far-field electrogram data generated by the endocardial surface are acquired by the MEA and fed into a multichannel recorder and amplifier system. Laplace's equation with boundary conditions can be used to describe how potentials at the endocardial boundary would appear at a remote location. The solution to the inverse Laplace's equation using the boundary element method would predict how a remotely detected signal by the EnSite Array™ would have appeared at its source, the endocardial border. The solution creates 3360 "virtual" endocardial electrograms making up the endocardial boundary.

The system also has a locater system to locate any conventional catheter in space relative to the EnSite Array™. Location is achieved by using a low-current, 5.68-kHz signal passed between the ablation tip and between the ring electrodes proximal and distal to the EnSite Array™. This is used to generate a more anatomically accurate endocardial model to plot the reconstructed endocardial electrograms. The locator signal is also used to display the position of the mapping catheter on the virtual endocardium during a study.

Limitations to the system include loss of accuracy of virtual electrograms if the endocardial surface is greater than 34 mm away from the balloon surface [12]. Large endocardial borders within a large volume may require MEA repositioning to collect adequate virtual electrogram data. This makes mapping of ventricular tachycardia in a large left ventricle potentially difficult. In addition, the EnSite Array™ has a volume of about 8–10 mL, and positioning of the MEA in small areas may limit the movement of the ablation catheter [13]. Low endocardial voltages may also be missed as it

may be too weak to be detected by the time the signal reaches the MEA. And lastly, during a 1:1 tachycardia, mapping in an area with simultaneous atrial and ventricular components such as atrioventricular nodal reentry tachycardia (AVNRT) may be difficult.

St. Jude Medical EnSite NavX™

The latest mapping technology to come to market is EnSite NavX™ by St. Jude Medical, which was first described by Ventura *et al.* in 2004 [14]. In a randomized study of 40 typical atrial flutter ablations comparing NavX™ to traditional fluoroscopy, the NavX™ system significantly reduced fluoroscopy time without significantly increasing procedural time. This mapping system allows the display of exact anatomical position of multiple conventional electrophysiology catheters in real time. In addition, the navigation system can be used with the EnSite Array™ catheter. The system has been used for mapping atrial and ventricular tachycardias [14,15].

The system includes three external orthogonal electrode pairs positioned on the body surface for catheter location [14,16,17] (Figure 1.4). One electrode pair is placed at the back of the neck above C3/4 and the medial upper left leg. The second electrode pair is placed on the left and right lateral thoracic cage close to T5/6. The third electrode pair is placed on the anterior and posterior chest at position T2. The six electrodes form three orthogonal axes with the heart at the center. A maximum of 64 electrodes (maximum 8 catheters) with up to 20 electrodes per catheter can be detected. A 5.68-kHz constant low-current locator signal is multiplexed with each pair of surface electrode to create a transthoracic electrical field. The potential

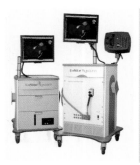 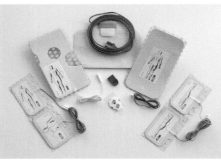

Figure 1.4 EnSite NavX™ navigation system (left) with external reference pads (right). (Courtesy of St. Jude Medical.)

difference between these electrode pairs and each catheter electrode is measured. A multiplex frequency of 93 Hz allows almost real-time navigation and visualization of catheter position. Any movement of the catheter causes a change in the measured voltage potential and impedance for each electrode. The potentials are defined with respect to a reference electrode. The reference electrode can be a surface electrode or an internally fixed electrode such as a coronary sinus catheter electrode. The position of the electrode can be determined to an accuracy of 0.6 mm. Electroanatomical mapping is obtained by manipulating a conventional mapping catheter throughout the heart cavity to generate a three-dimensional endocardial border. An endocardial surface geometry can be generated in a short period of time.

One potential limitation to the EnSite NavX™ system similar to the CARTO™ system is that it requires a stable rhythm as mapping is done sequentially on a point-by-point and beat-to-beat basis. However, unlike CARTO™, electrograms from multiple poles of a catheter may be recorded simultaneously. The EnSite NavX™ has recently released a software version that allows integration with CT or MRI. Adding this will undoubtedly increase the utility of this mapping system in the ablation of atrial fibrillation and potentially ventricular tachycardia as well.

Boston Scientific RPM™ Realtime Position Management

The RPM™ Realtime Position Management by Boston Scientific (Natick, MA) was first used and described by de Groot *et al.* in 2000 [18]. In that study, 30 patients referred for radiofrequency catheter ablation used the RPM™ system to map and track the position of the ablation catheter relative to two reference catheters with good success. The Boston Scientific RPM™ Realtime Position Management system is the first mapping system to use the technique of ultrasound ranging for mapping. The system uses an internal reference system that removes the need for skin electrodes or patches as well as minimizes the impact of respiratory variations and patient movement. The system has been validated in both atrial and ventricular tachycardia [18,19].

The navigation and mapping system includes an acquisition module and an ultrasound transmitter/receiver unit connected to a SPARC 20 computer (Sun Microsystems, Palo Alto, CA). The system can simultaneously process seven position management catheters, 24 bipolar/48 unipolar electrograms, a 12-lead ECG, and 2 pressure signals. The intracardiac part consists of a series of transmitters and receivers of ultrasound pulses on reference catheters. The time delay between transmitters and receivers is proportional to the distance between the transducers assuming a speed of sound in the blood of 1550 m/s. The time and distance information is transmitted back to the computer for real-time display. The catheter positions are used to reconstruct a three-dimensional endocardial geometry. There are three catheters, two reference catheters, and one mapping/ablation catheter. The reference catheters are 6-Fr multipolar catheters, and the first reference catheter is usually positioned in the right ventricle and the second reference catheter can be positioned in the right appendage, lateral right atrium, or the coronary sinus. For mapping/ablation, a 7-Fr, 4-mm-tip bidirectional steerable ablation catheter is used. The reference catheters are equipped with four ultrasound transducers whereas the ablation catheter only has three. The right atrial reference catheter contains nine 1-mm ring electrodes and one 2-mm tip electrode with 1-mm interelectrode distance. The right ventricular reference catheter contains three 1-mm ring electrodes and one 4-mm tip electrode. The ultrasound transmitter sends a continuous cycle of ultrasound pulses at 558.5 kHz to the transducers of the reference and ablation catheters. The electroanatomic mapping of the heart is generated by manipulation of the mapping catheter along the endocardial surface.

A limitation to this system is the need of at least three catheters to provide internal reference. As the localizing technology uses ultrasound frequency, the use of intracardiac echocardiography may be limited. In addition, the catheters are proprietary single-use catheters made by Boston Scientific.

Future direction of electroanatomic mapping

Electroanatomical mapping is increasingly being used for all kinds of ablation procedures. The technology including better mapping and visualization has improved significantly over the past few years.

In addition, advancements in integration with CT and MRI data sets are improving rapidly. Future advancements may include electroanatomical map integration with intracardiac echocardiogram or three-dimensional fluoroscopy.

References

1. Ben-Haim, S.A., D. Osadchy, I. Schuster, *et al.*, Nonfluoroscopic, *in vivo* navigation and mapping technology. *Nat Med*, 1996. **2**(12): p. 1393–5.

2. Nademanee, K. and E.M. Kosar, A nonfluoroscopic catheter-based mapping technique to ablate focal ventricular tachycardia. *Pacing Clin Electrophysiol*, 1998. **21**(7): p. 1442–7.

3. Khongphatthanayothin, A., E. Kosar, and K. Nademanee, Nonfluoroscopic three-dimensional mapping for arrhythmia ablation: tool or toy? *J Cardiovasc Electrophysiol*, 2000. **11**(3): p. 239–43.

4. Nakagawa, H. and W.M. Jackman, Use of a three-dimensional, nonfluoroscopic mapping system for catheter ablation of typical atrial flutter. *Pacing Clin Electrophysiol*, 1998. **21**(6): p. 1279–86.

5. Willems, S., C.Weiss, R. Ventura, *et al.*, Catheter ablation of atrial flutter guided by electroanatomic mapping (CARTO): a randomized comparison to the conventional approach. *J Cardiovasc Electrophysiol*, 2000. **11**(11): p. 1223–30.

6. Marchlinski, F.E., D.J. Callans, C.D. Gottlieb, and E. Zado, Linear ablation lesions for control of unmappable ventricular tachycardia in patients with ischemic and nonischemic cardiomyopathy. *Circulation*, 2000. **101**(11): p. 1288–96.

7. Gepstein, L., G. Hayam, and S.A. Ben-Haim, A novel method for nonfluoroscopic catheter-based electroanatomical mapping of the heart. *In vitro* and *in vivo* accuracy results. *Circulation*, 1997. **95**(6): p. 1611–22.

8. Tops, L.F., J.J. Bax , K. Zeppenfeld, *et al.*, Fusion of multislice computed tomography imaging with three-dimensional electroanatomic mapping to guide radiofrequency catheter ablation procedures. *Heart Rhythm*, 2005. **2**(10): p. 1076–81.

9. Dong, J., T. Dickfeld, D. Dalal, et al., Initial experience in the use of integrated electroanatomic mapping with three-dimensional MR/CT images to guide catheter ablation of atrial fibrillation. *J Cardiovasc Electrophysiol*, 2006. **17**(5): p. 459–66.

10. Verma, A., N. Marrouche, and A. Natale, Novel method to integrate three-dimensional computed tomographic images of the left atrium with real-time electroanatomic mapping. *J Cardiovasc Electrophysiol*, 2004. **15**(8): p. 968.

11. Fahmy, T.S., H. Mlcochova, O.M. Wazni, *et al.*, Intracardiac echo-guided image integration: optimizing strategies for registration. *J Cardiovasc Electrophysiol*, 2007. **18**(3): p. 276–82.

12. Schilling, R.J., N.S. Peters, and D.W. Davies, Simultaneous endocardial mapping in the human left ventricle using a noncontact catheter: comparison of contact and reconstructed electrograms during sinus rhythm. *Circulation*, 1998. **98**(9): p. 887–98.

13. Packer, D.L., Three-dimensional mapping in interventional electrophysiology: techniques and technology. *J Cardiovasc Electrophysiol*, 2005. **16**(10): p. 1110–6.

14. Ventura, R., T. Rostock, H.U. Klemm, *et al.*, Catheter ablation of common-type atrial flutter guided by three-dimensional right atrial geometry reconstruction and catheter tracking using cutaneous patches: a randomized prospective study. *J Cardiovasc Electrophysiol*, 2004. **15**(10): p. 1157–61.

15. Earley, M.J., R. Showkathali, M. Alzetani, *et al.*, Radiofrequency ablation of arrhythmias guided by non-fluoroscopic catheter location: a prospective randomized trial. *Eur Heart J*, 2006. **27**(10): p. 1223–9.

16. Krum, D., A. Goel, J. Hauck, *et al.*, Catheter location, tracking, cardiac chamber geometry creation, and ablation using cutaneous patches. *J Interv Card Electrophysiol*, 2005. **12**(1): p. 17–22.

17. Novak, P.G., L. Macle, B. Thibault, and P.G. Guerra, Enhanced left atrial mapping using digitally synchronized NavX three-dimensional nonfluoroscopic mapping and high-resolution computed tomographic imaging for catheter ablation of atrial fibrillation. *Heart Rhythm*, 2004. **1**(4): p. 521–2.

18. de Groot, N.M., M. Bootsma, E.T. van der Velde, and M.J. Schalij, Three-dimensional catheter positioning during radiofrequency ablation in patients: first application of a real-time position management system. *J Cardiovasc Electrophysiol*, 2000. **11**(11): p. 1183–92.

19. Schreieck, J., G. Ndrepepa, B. Zrenner, et al., Radiofrequency ablation of cardiac arrhythmias using a three-dimensional real-time position management and mapping system. *Pacing Clin Electrophysiol*, 2002. **25**(12): p. 1699–707.

CHAPTER 2

Electroanatomical mapping for supraventricular tachycardias

Pirooz Mofrad, MD, *Amin Al-Ahmad*, MD, *& Andrea Natale*, MD

Introduction

Three-dimensional electroanatomic mapping technologies are being increasingly utilized for the catheter ablation of arrhythmias. These computerized mapping systems allow for the creation of a three-dimensional map of cardiac chambers while obtaining information on tissue voltage and local electrogram timing with respect to a reference. The ability to generate relatively high-density voltage maps have allowed for the identification of areas of presumed scar, or low-voltage, that may be critical in the development of reentry. Identification of these areas is thus useful to identify candidate areas that may be a critical isthmus site for reentry even in the absence of inducible arrhythmias. In addition, complete cardiac-cycle activation mapping during both reentrant and automatic tachyarrhythmias allows for the identification of the site of focal activation and the visualization of complete reentrant loops utilized by reentrant tachycardias [1].

The use of electroanatomical mapping systems has had a major impact on anatomically guided approaches to radiofrequency (RF) ablation. The clinical utility of these systems includes assisting in creating lesion sets by reconstructing a three-dimensional view of the chamber of interest and allowing the visualization on the reconstructed anatomy of any previous ablation lesions, thus helping in the goal of creating contiguous lesions and identifying areas that were not adequately ablated. In addition, sites with interesting electrograms,

Electroanatomical Mapping, 1st edition. Edited by A. Al-Ahmad, D. Callans, H. Hsia and A. Natale. © 2008 Blackwell Publishing, ISBN: 9781405157025.

electrical unexcitability, and specific anatomic structures can be tagged, allowing for ease of return of the mapping catheters to these previous positions and avoidance of critical areas such as the conduction system.

Previous studies have evaluated the utility of electroanatomical mapping systems in a myriad of atrial tachyarrhythmias including atrial flutter, atrial fibrillation, focal atrial tachycardias, atrioventricular reciprocating tachycardia (AVRT), and atrioventricular nodal reentry tachycardia (AVNRT). Although electroanatomic mapping systems for catheter ablation procedures may not consistently reduce procedural duration, they have been shown to reduce fluoroscopy time and radiation dose, as well as reduce the number of catheters that may be utilized [2]. In addition, electroanatomic mapping systems have aided in the understanding of the propagation of normal sinus impulses, interatrial conduction, and impulse propagation of left- and right-sided atrial tachycardias, facilitating our understanding of not only interatrial conduction patterns but also how they relate to the surface 12-lead P-wave morphology serving to link the known anatomic structure to electrical activity [3].

Focal atrial tachycardia

Although focal atrial tachycardias commonly cluster at anatomical structures such as the crista terminalis, the tricuspid and mitral annulus, the pulmonary veins (PVs), and the atrial appendages, intracardiac mapping of these tachycardias can be a challenge and is aided by the use of electroanatomical mapping systems [4]. Multiple algorithms exist that utilize P-wave morphology on 12-lead

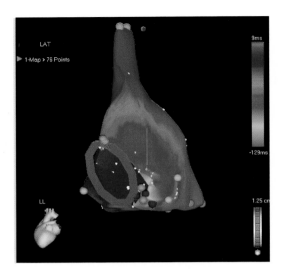

Figure 2.1 Three-dimensional electroanatomic map using Biosense CARTO™ of patient with recurrent symptomatic SVT. Electrophysiology (EP) study along with activation map reveals focal atrial tachycardia (FAT) with earliest focal activation at the coronary sinus ostium (CS). Deliver of RF energy at this site abolished the tachycardia.

electrocardiograms to help localize the origin of these tachycardias; despite these algorithms, precise localization can only be done with mapping catheters and is greatly aided with the use of electroanatomical mapping [5–8]. The ability to integrate anatomical tags such as valvular points and areas of interest such as areas of scar or fractionated electrograms is also useful in generating a complete map that can aid in the localization of the earliest site of activation and best potential site for delivery of ablation lesions [9] (Figure 2.1). High-resolution visualization of endocardial impulse propagation and activation during focal atrial tachycardias, displayed on a three-dimensional recreated anatomical shell via electroanatomical mapping systems, has facilitated our understanding and ablation of focal atrial tachycardia [10–13].

Noncontact mapping systems (EnSite 3000, Endocardial Solutions, Inc, St. Paul, MN) have been used to facilitate the mapping of focal atrial tachycardia by generating over 3000 virtual unipolar electrograms on a reconstructed three-dimensional endocardial shell [14,15]. High-density isopotential maps depict endocardial activation and wave front propagation. One advantage of this technology is that transient nonsustained atrial tachyarrhythmias

can be easily and rapidly localized. In a study by Seidl *et al.*, 25 ectopic atrial tachycardias were identified in 22 patients with noncontact mapping used to identify the site of earliest endocardial activation [14]. The success rate using this approach was 92%, with all transient atrial tachycardias successfully ablated.

Natale demonstrated the ability to rapidly map and ablate both right and left ectopic atrial tachycardias using the Biosense CARTO™ system [16]. In the 24 patients included in this study, 13 atrial tachycardias were mapped to the left atrium and 16 originated from the right atrium. Earliest sites of endocardial activation were targeted, with a predominance of clustering along the crista terminalis and PVs. A mean of four RF applications were necessary with the average fluoroscopy time required to generate the activation maps and perform the ablation of 7 min. The high success rate noted in this early study (one patient required repeat ablation with the rest remaining symptom-free) underscored the strength of the system in allowing the operator to renavigate the mapping electrode to the exact same locations on the map, along with the reconstruction of a three-dimensional activation and geometry of the atrial chambers.

The use of three-dimensional electroanatomical mapping for sinus node modification in the treatment of inappropriate sinus tachycardia has also been reported [17,18]. In a study of 35 patients by Marrouche, successful mapping of the sinus node area with the Biosense CARTO™ system was performed and remapping of the earliest site of endocardial activation after ablation was facilitated by the use of electroanatomical mapping [17]. Noncontact mapping systems have been used in limited, small nonrandomized studies for the ablation of inappropriate sinus tachycardia with the advantage of continuous real-time and updated endocardial activation maps [19,20].

Atrioventricular nodal reentrant tachycardia and atrioventricular reciprocating tachycardia

AVNRT has been a focus of extensive research with delineation of the anatomic triangle of Koch and the realization of the numerous anterior and posterior inputs into the atrioventricular (AV) node that play an important role in the physiology of this arrhythmia.

Cooke and Wilber described their initial experience in 14 patients with an anatomical approach utilizing the Biosense CARTO™ system to create a high-density electroanatomical map of the triangle of Koch in normal sinus rhythm to facilitate slow pathway modification [21]. In this study, electroanatomical mapping of the triangle of Koch could be performed in less than 30 min, with anatomic areas being tagged such as the coronary sinus ostium, the tricuspid annulus, and the "His cluster." Utilizing this technique, the authors were able to limit their delivery of RF energy to a level below 1 cm from the His cluster, theoretically reducing the possibility of damage to the AV node and complete heart block. In this study, a median of two RF energy pulses was necessary to eliminate inducible AVNRT with no cases of heart block. Figure 2.2 is a representative St. Jude NavX electroanatomic map of the right atrium during AVNRT, with earliest atrial retrograde activation noted at the His.

In addition, electroanatomic mapping of the triangle of Koch may facilitate the understanding of complex anatomy in postsurgical, congenital, and dilated right atriums where the distance and orientation between the coronary sinus ostium and His cluster may be altered. In a recent case described by Khairy et al., a patient with a surgically repaired partial AV canal defect underwent a successful slow pathway modification for AVNRT

with the assistance of the EnSite NavX system [22]. Three-dimensional electroanatomic mapping of the triangle of Koch facilitated delineation of the inverted inputs to the AV node with successful ablation of the slow pathway input superior to the His bundle.

Further benefits of utilizing electroanatomical mapping for AVNRT include a reduction in fluoroscopic time utilizing the Biosense CARTO™ system compared with the traditional fluoroscopy [23,24]. Kopelman et al. performed a prospective randomized trial with enrollment of 20 consecutive patients comparing conventional fluoroscopic slow pathway modification to electroanatomical guided approach utilizing the Biosense CARTO™ system with respect to acute procedural success, fluoroscopic and procedural time, and total energy delivery [24]. Acute procedural success was 100% in both groups. However, ablation, fluoroscopic exposure, and procedure time were all reduced in the electroanatomic mapping group with an average of 2.7 RF energy pulses compared with 5 in the conventional fluoroscopic arm.

The utility of using three-dimensional electroanatomic mapping systems for localizing the insertion of accessory pathways for catheter ablation has been investigated in limited studies [2,25–27]. The benefits of mapping systems included the ability to tag interesting sites, navigate to previously investigated areas, and to define the extent of the AV node to reduce inadvertent injury. In addition, limited

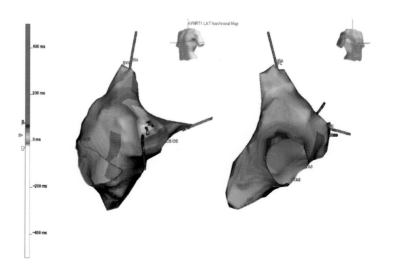

Figure 2.2. Three-dimensional electroanatomic map of activation during AVNRT created by NavX. Note earliest retrograde atrial activation at the His bundle.

studies suggest a reduction of total fluoroscopic time with the use of electroanatomic mapping systems [2,26]. Electroanatomic mapping systems can also be useful in cases of failed catheter ablation. In a study by Gonzalez-Torrecilla *et al.*, 17 patients with accessory pathways who had failed an average of two previous conventional procedures underwent three-dimensional electroanatomic mapping guided ablation (with the Biosense CARTO™ system) with a 94% success rate (1 failure), with no recurrences during a mean follow-up of 16 ± 15 months [27]. Successful ablations of anatomically challenging accessory pathways associated with either coronary sinus diverticuli or Epstein's anomaly have been described in the literature with the assistance of three-dimensional electroanatomic mapping systems [28–30].

In summary, three-dimensional electroanatomical mapping of AVNRT and AVRT may not improve the already high efficacy of these ablations, but it may reduce fluoroscopy time, catalogue previous delivered ablation lesions, and be an aid in cases with unique or complex anatomy.

Macroreentrant atrial tachycardias

Typical and reverse typical atrial flutter

Clockwise and counterclockwise cavotricuspid isthmus-dependent atrial flutter is a well-characterized right atrial macroreentrant tachyarrhythmia that can be eliminated by linear ablation along the cavotricuspid isthmus (CTI) [31] (Figure 2.3).

Three-dimensional electroanatomic mapping has proven beneficial in reducing fluoroscopic time for this procedure [32–35]. Three-dimensional electroanatomical mapping has facilitated our understanding of the complex anatomy of the cavotricuspid isthmus CTI, reconstructing anatomic variation such as the presence of pouches, and gaining insight as to the length and concavity of the isthmus that could potentially assist in adequate delivery of linear ablation lesions [35,36]. In a study by Chang *et al.*, correlation of the anatomy of the CTI between electroanatomic mapping (using St. Jude NavX system) and right atrial angiography was investigated, with the examination of CTI characteristics that predicted outcomes of RF ablation [36]. Three-dimensional electroanatomic mapping images of the CTI correlated well with

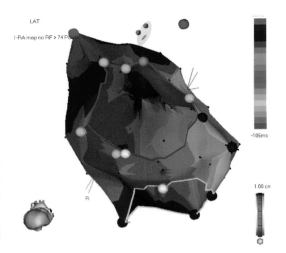

Figure 2.3 Endocardial activation map with the Biosense CARTO™ system in patient with typical atrial flutter. Note the early-meets-late wave front consistent with counterclockwise typical atrial flutter.

angiographic results for the CTI length, depth (in cases of concavity), and the presence and dimensions of CTI pouches. The patients with pouch-type CTI had longer ablation, procedural, and fluoroscopic times with a larger number of RF applications as well, but no clinical recurrences. In comparison, a group of 50 patients who served as a control group underwent conventional mapping and ablation under fluoroscopy. In this group, the ablation, fluoroscopy, and procedural times were longer than in the image-guided group. In addition, the control group had a larger number of RF applications and three clinical recurrences during the mean follow-up period of 11 ± 4 months.

Although there is no evidence from randomized trials that ablation time is reduced using electroanatomical mapping, several studies have examined the utility of this technology for the treatment of atrial flutter. Kottkamp *et al.* prospectively randomized a total of 50 patients to conventional fluoroscopic-directed isthmus ablation or electroanatomic mapping utilizing the Biosense CARTO™ system [32]. Complete isthmus block was achieved in over 94% of the patients with the overall fluoroscopic time reduced from an average of 22 min in the fluoroscopic-directed group to 3.9 min in the electroanatomical group. Willems *et al.* produced similar findings in a randomized prospective trial of fluoroscopy versus electroanatomical mapping in 80 consecutive patients undergoing ablation for antiarrhythmic therapy refractory typical atrial flutter with similar efficacy and recurrence rates, and a reduction in overall fluoroscopic time from a mean of 29.2 min in the standard fluoroscopy group as compared with 7.7 min in the electroanatomical mapping group [33].

Despite its well-defined isthmus, recurrence of atrial flutter postablation is possible. Localization of gaps allowing for the resumption of electrical conduction can be performed with conventional electrogram mapping techniques. High-density electroanatomical mapping of the activation through an incomplete isthmus ablation line can be performed to locate these electrical gaps, further facilitating their target for repeat ablation [37,38]. In a study by Sra *et al.*, 12 patients with recurrent typical atrial flutter underwent detailed voltage, activation, and propagation mapping of the CTI (utilizing Biosense CARTO™ system) with precise identification of gaps in all 12 patients. After application of RF energy at these gap sites, atrial flutter was eliminated in all of the 12 patients, confirmed by noninducibility and bidirectional conduction block along the isthmus [38]. Only one recurrence was noted after a mean follow-up of greater than 14 months. Figure 2.4 shows identification of a gap along the CTI in a patient with recurrent atrial flutter using the Endocardial Solutions ESI system. This patient was successfully treated with a single ablation lesion at the site of the gap. The use of electroanatomical mapping systems for the localization of gaps along the lesion line in the CTI is a useful technique,

especially in cases of clinical recurrence of atrial flutter.

Electroanatomic mapping systems may reduce fluoroscopy time and provide guidance for the placement and monitoring of a linear lesion set along the CTI, but it cannot supplant or eliminate the need for basic electrophysiology maneuvers to confirm isthmus-dependent atrial flutter. It is a useful tool for the localization of linear gaps in recurrent atrial flutter, after conventional techniques, including entrainment mapping after performed.

Atypical intraatrial reentrant tachyarrhythmias

Conventional mapping and ablation techniques of atypical atrial flutters that can arise are a result of atrial scar such as patients with surgically corrected congenital heart disease can be challenging. Macroreentrant atrial tachycardias can use, as their critical isthmus, zones of slow conduction within a scar or between an anatomical boundary and an incisional scar. Three-dimensional electroanatomic mapping systems are helpful in creating high-density atrial endocardial voltage and activation maps to identify these sites of prior scar and for tagging of anatomic structures, allowing for visualization of the zones of slow conduction responsible for serving as the critical isthmus that provides for the perpetuation of these tachyarrhythmias [39–44].

Postincisional intraatrial reentrant tachycardias can be particularly difficult to map using conventional fluoroscopic techniques, especially in the setting of congenital or structural heart disease where normal anatomic structures are displaced.

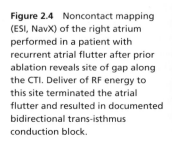

Figure 2.4 Noncontact mapping (ESI, NavX) of the right atrium performed in a patient with recurrent atrial flutter after prior ablation reveals site of gap along the CTI. Deliver of RF energy to this site terminated the atrial flutter and resulted in documented bidirectional trans-isthmus conduction block.

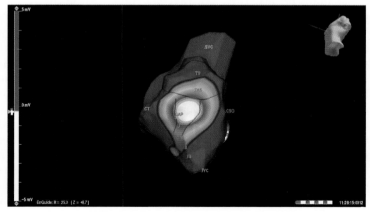

Shah *et al.* used the Biosense CARTO™ system to establish the existence of dual-loop intraatrial reentrant circuits in five consecutive patients with drug-resistant atrial tachyarrhythmia after surgical closure of ostium secundum atrial septal defects [45]. Marrouche *et al.* utilized the Biosense CARTO™ system to describe the existence of a macroreentrant left septal atrial flutter, typically occurring after the initiation of antiarrhythmic drug therapy for atrial fibrillation [46]. In addition to clearly delineating sites of surgical endocardial scar with voltage mapping, three-dimensional electroanatomical mapping can also allow for rapid distinction between focal peri-incisional atrial tachycardias versus intraatrial reentrant tachyarrhythmias in postoperative patients. In a study by Reithmann *et al.*, 10 postsurgical patients underwent three-dimensional electroanatomical mapping for 13 incisional atrial tachycardias [47]. Activation mapping with the Biosense CARTO™ system during the atrial tachycardias quickly differentiated the 10 macroreentrant rhythms from the focal atrial tachycardia, with a continuous atrial activation and early-meets-late pattern versus a radial centrifugal pattern of activation in all directions from an earliest endocardial site, respectively. The three-dimensional electroanatomical mapping systems have also been useful in improving our understanding and localization of incisional atrial tachycardia's (AT) postorthotopic heart transplantation with donor–recipient atrial tachyarrhythmias [48].

Atrial fibrillation

The role of catheter ablation for atrial fibrillation has continued to expand over the past several years. Outcomes for ablation have also continued to improve such that ablation for atrial fibrillation (AF) is considered earlier in the treatment algorithm of patients with atrial fibrillation [49]. Three-dimensional electroanatomical mapping systems have been utilized extensively for this procedure. Three-dimensional electroanatomical mapping has assisted catheter manipulation within the atria by facilitating anatomically guided delivery of linear ablation sets around the PVs and within the atria [50–52].

Continued advancements in merging reconstructed anatomic intracardiac images via preprocedural CT and MRI scans with an intraoperative electroanatomic endocardial map may prove to have an impact on procedural success and safety. Validation of the first clinically available image integration system for catheter ablation (CartoMerge), merging Biosense CARTO™ system derived endocardial maps and CT images with necropsy data, resulted in an accuracy of less than 3 mm in all four cardiac chambers [53]. In a nonrandomized study by Kistler *et al.*, CT integration into the electroanatomic mapping system during catheter ablation for atrial fibrillation was associated with reduced fluoroscopy times, arrhythmia recurrence, and increased restoration of sinus rhythm [54]. The display of detailed left atrial geometry, including the three-dimensional location and number of PVs and anatomic variants, may theoretically aid in individualizing tailored catheter ablation procedures with improvements in efficacy and safety [55,56]. In addition, information gleaned from three-dimensional electroanatomic mapping, in particular the burden of left atrial scar, has been demonstrated to be predictive of PV isolation procedural failure with significantly higher atrial fibrillation recurrence rates [57]. Finally, caution must be directed in the registration and integration process with CartoMerge, so as to avoid large errors. There is evidence that a smaller mean error results for the image integration process if posterior intracardiac landmark points are selected, as opposed to anterior structures [58].

Large circumferential isolation lesion sets, if incomplete, may favor the development of postablation left-sided atypical atrial flutters. Evidence from single-center studies support the creation of additional linear lesion sets, including a CTI line, mitral isthmus line (connecting the mitral isthmus and the left inferior pulmonary vein (PV)), and posterior superior line connecting the contralateral PVs, in order to reduce postablation atrial tachyarrhythmias [59–61]. However, as with any linear lesion, incomplete ablation lines allows for gaps that promote the development of incessant left-sided atypical atrial flutter. Similar issues remain in the postsurgical cohort of patients who undergo direct visual endocardial or epicardial linear lesion set delivery. Resumption of conduction and resultant electrical gaps in the linear lesion sets that result in atypical postoperative left atrial flutters have been reported, with three-dimensional electroanatomical mapping successfully utilized to locate these gaps and deliver RF energy to terminate the arrhythmia [62].

Electrical isolation of the pulmonary veins using three-dimensional electroanatomical mapping can reduce fluoroscopic exposure and procedural time. Estner *et al.* evaluated the feasibility of performing segmental PV isolations guided by the St. Jude Medical NavX™ system versus fluoroscopic guidance in a cohort of 64 patients [63]. PV mapping and ablation with the assistance of a circular mapping catheter yielded similar primary success rates for PV isolation, with the St. Jude Medical NavX™ system-guided procedures showing a significant reduction in fluoroscopic (75.8 min vs. 38.9 min) and procedural time (237.7 min vs. 188.6 min). Three-dimensional electroanatomical mapping in conjunction with impedance mapping (rise in impedance of > 4 ohms) can facilitate the identification of the LA–PV transitional zone and therefore a suitable and safe site for delivery of RF energy during PV isolation with a low risk of PV stenosis [64].

Integration of data regarding esophageal position during three-dimensional electroanatomical-mapping-guided atrial fibrillation ablations can potentially serve to avoid and limit injury to the esophagus during left atrial posterior ablations. The esophagus can be tagged and integrated into either the St. Jude Medical NavX™ system or the Biosense CARTO™ system with real-time visualization of the course and position of the esophagus in relation to the ablation catheter and the LA and PVs [65–67]. Titration of energy or avoidance of delivery of a lesion set to high-risk areas can be performed. The integration of three-dimensional electroanatomical mapping systems for catheter ablation of atrial fibrillation has proven to be invaluable, allowing for improvement in delivery of a linear lesion set and possibly improving the efficacy of PV isolation and reducing the procedural time.

More recently, the use of noncontact mapping electrodes to define the location of dominant frequencies in atrial fibrillation in the left atrium both before and after ablation, has improved our understanding of the substrate for the initiation and maintenance of atrial fibrillation [68,69].

Conclusion

Three-dimensional electroanatomical mapping systems have facilitated our treatment and understanding of the mechanisms operating in complex arrhythmias. Electroanatomic mapping systems have been proven to reduce fluoroscopic time, procedural time, and may improve ablation success in supraventricular tachyarrhythmias (SVTs). The creation of linear ablation lines and the accurate return of the catheter to previous ablation sites are invaluable advantages gained by the use of these systems. The use of electroanatomic mapping in the ablation of many SVTs may not be necessary, but its utility in cataloging and tagging interesting endocardial sites and ablation lesions, along with its construction and identification of low-voltage scar sites, facilitates our understanding of arrhythmia propagation and perpetuation.

References

1. Veranasi, S., A. Dhala, Z. Blanck, S. Deshpande, M. Akhtar, J. Sra, Electroanatomic mapping for radiofrequency ablation of cardiac arrhythmias. *JCE*, April 1999; **10**: 538–44.

2. Sporton, S.C., M.J. Earley, A.W. Nathan, R.J. Schilling. Electroanatomic versus fluoroscopic mapping for catheter ablation procedures: a prospective randomized study. *J. Cardiovasc. Electrophysiol.*, March 2004; **15**: 310–15.

3. De, P.R., S.Y. Ho, J.A. Salerno-Uriarte, M. Tritto, G. Spadacini, Electroanatomic analysis of sinus impulse propagation in normal human atria. *JCE*, January 2002; **13**: 1–10.

4. Roberts-Thomson, K.C., P.M. Kistler, J.M. Kalman, Focal atrial tachycardia I: clinical features, diagnosis, mechanisms, and anatomic location. *PACE*, 2006; **29**: 643–52.

5. Tada, H, A. Nogami, S. Naito, *et al.* Simple electrocardiographic criteria for identifying the site of origin of focal right atrial tachycardia. *PACE*, 1998; **21**[Pt. II]: 2431–9.

6. Kistler, P.M., K.C. Roberts-Thomson, H.M. Haqqani, *et al.* P-wave morphology in focal atrial tachycardia. *JACC*, 2006; **48**: 1010–17.

7. Tang, C.W., M.M. Scheinman, G.F. Van Hare, *et al.* Use of p wave configuration during atrial tachycardia to predict site of origin. *JACC*, 1995; **26**: 1315–24.

8. Rajawat, Y.S., E.P. Gerstenfeld, V.V. Patel, S. Dixit, D.J. Callans, FE Marchilinski. ECG criteria for localizing the pulmonary vein origin of spontaneous atrial premature complexes: validation using intracardiac recordings. *PACE*, 2004; **27**: 182–8.

9. Kottkamp, H, G. Hindricks, G. Breithardt, M. Borggrefe. Three-dimensional electromagnetic catheter technology: electroanatomical mapping of the right atrium and ablation of ectopic atrial tachycardia. *J. Cardiovasc. Electrophysiol.*, December 1997; **8**(12): 1332–7.

10. Cavaco, D., Adragao, P., Morgado, F., *et al.* Electroanatomical mapping and ablation of atrial tachycardias with

the CARTO system. *Rev. Port. Cardiol.*, April 2002; **21**(4): 407–18.

11. Hoffmann, E., P. Nimmermann, C. Reithmann, F. Elser, T. Remp, G. Steinbeck. New mapping technology for atrial tachycardias. *J. Interv. Card. Electrophysiol.*, January 2000; **4**(Suppl 1): 117–20.

12. Hoffmann, E., C. Reithmann, P. Nimmermann, *et al.* Clinical experience with electroanatomic mapping of ectopic atrial tachycardia. *PACE*, 2002; **25**: 49–56.

13. Marchlinski, F. Magnetic electroanatomical mapping for ablation of focal atrial tachycardias. *PACE*, August 1998; **21**(8): 1621–35.

14. Seidl, K., H. Schwacke, M. Rameken, A. Drogemuller, G. Beatty, J. Senges. Noncontact mapping of ectopic atrial tachycardias: different characteristics of isopotential maps and unipolar electrogram. *PACE*, 2003; **26** [Pt I]: 16–25.

15. Higa, S., C.T. Tai, Y.J. Lin, *et al.* Focal atrial tachycardia: new insight from noncontact mapping and catheter ablation. *Circulation*, 2004; **109**: 84–91.

16. Natale, A. Ablation of right and left ectopic atrial tachycardias using a three-dimensional nonfluoroscopic mapping system. *Am. J. Cardiol.*, October 1998; **82**: 989–92.

17. Marrouche, F. Nassir. Three-dimensional nonfluoroscopic mapping and ablation of inappropriate sinus tachycardia. *JACC*, 2002; **39**: 1046–54.

18. Leonelli, F., M. Richey, S. Beheiry, K. Rajkovich, A. Natale. Tridimensional mapping: guided modification of the sinus node. *J. Cardiovasc. Electrophysiol.*, November 1998; **9**: 1214–17.

19. Lin, D., F. Garcia, J. Jacobson, *et al.* Use of noncontact mapping and saline-cooled ablation catheter for sinus node modification in medically refractory inappropriate sinus tachycardia. *PACE*, 2007; **30**: 236–42.

20. Bonhomme, C.E., F.T. Deger, J. Schultz, S.S. Hsu. Radiofrequency catheter ablation using non-contact mapping for inappropriate sinus tachycardia. *J. Interv. Card. Electrophysiol.*, 2004; **10**: 159–63.

21. Cooke, P.A., D.J. Wilber. Radiofrequency catheter ablation of atrioventricular nodal reentry tachycardia utilizing nonfluoroscopic electroanatomical mapping. *PACE*, 1998; **21**: 1802–9.

22. Khairy, P., L.A. Mercier, A. Dore, M. Dubuc. Partial atrioventricular canal defect with inverted atrioventricular nodal input into an inferiorly displaced atrioventricular node. *Heart Rhythm*, 2007; **4**(3): 355–8.

23. Khongphatthanayothin, A., E. Kosar, K. Nademanee. Nonfluoroscopic three-dimensional mapping for arrhythmia ablation tool or toy? *J. Cardiovasc. Electrophysiol.*, March 2000; **11**(3): 239–43.

24. Kopelman, H.A., S.P. Prater, F. Tondato, N.A. Chronos, N.S. Peters, Slow pathway catheter ablation of atrioventricular nodal re-entrant tachycardia guided by electro-

anatomical mapping: a randomized comparison to the conventional approach. *Europace*, 2003; **5**: 171–4.

25. Worley, S.J. Use of real-time three-dimensional magnetic navigation system for radiofrequency ablation of accessory pathways. *PACE*, 1998; **21**: 1636–45.

26. Drago, F., M.S. Silvetti, A. Di Pino, G Grutter, M Bevilacqua, S Leibovich. Exclusion of fluoroscopy during ablation treatment of right accessory pathway in children. *J. Cardiovasc. Electrophysiol.*, 2002; **13**: 778–82.

27. Gonzalez-Torrecilla, E., A. Arenal, F. Atienza, J Almendral. Utility of nonfluoroscopic three-dimensional electroanatomical mapping in accessory pathways with prior unsuccessful ablation techniques. *Am. J. Cardiol.*, 2005; **96**: 564–9.

28. Ai T., S. Ikeguchi, M. Watanuki, *et al.* Successful radiofrequency current catheter ablation of accessory atrioventricular pathway in Ebstein's anomaly using electroanatomic mapping. *PACE*, 2002; **25**: 374–5.

29. Boulos, M., L. Gepstein. Electroanatomical mapping and radiofrequency ablation of an accessory pathway associated with a large aneurysm of the coronary sinus. *Europace*, 2004; **6**: 608–12.

30. Eckardt, L., G. Monnig, K. Wasmer, G. Breithardt. A NavX guided cryoablation of an accessory pathway in a large coronary sinus diverticulum. *J. Cardiovasc. Electrophysiol.*, 2005; **16**(2): 233–4.

31. Kirkorian, G., E. Moncada, P. Chevalier, *et al.* Radiofrequency ablation of atrial flutter—efficacy of an anatomically guided approach. *Circulation*, 1994; **90**: 2804–14..

32. Kottkamp, H., B. Hugl, B. Krauss, *et al.* Electromagnetic versus fluoroscopic mapping of the inferior isthmus for ablation typical atrial flutter—a prospective randomized study. *Circulation*, 2000; **102**: 2082–6.

33. Willems, S., C. Weiss, R. Ventura, *et al.* Catheter ablation of atrial flutter guided by electroanatomic mapping (CARTO): a randomized comparison to the conventional approach. *J. Cardiovasc. Electrophysiol.*, November 2000; **11**: 1223–30.

34. Leonelli, F.M., G. Tomassoni, M. Richey, A. Natale. Usefulness of three-dimensional non-fluoroscopic mapping in the ablation of typical atrial flutter. *Ital. Heart J.*, 2002; **3**(6): 360–5.

35. Ventura, R., T. Rostock, H.U. Klemm, *et al.* Catheter ablation of common-type atrial flutter guided by three-dimensional right atrial geometry reconstruction and catheter tracking using cutaneous patches: a randomized prospective study. *J. Cardiovasc. Electrophysiol.*, October 2004; **15**: 1157–61.

36. Chang, S., C. Tai, Y. Lin, *et al.* The electroanatomic characteristics of the cavotricuspid isthmus: implications for the catheter ablation of atrial flutter. *J. Cardiovasc. Electrophysiol.*, January 2007; **18**: 18–22.

37. Shah, D., M. Haissaguerre, P. Jais, A. Takahashi, M Hocini, J Clementy. High-density mapping of activation through an incomplete isthmus ablation line. *Circulation*, 1999; **99**: 211–5.

38. Sra, J., A. Bhatia, A. Dhala, *et al.* Electroanatomic mapping to identify breakthrough sites in recurrent typical human flutter. *PACE*, 2000; **23**[Pt 1]: 1479–92.

39. Kall, J.G., D.S. Rubenstein, D.E. Kopp, Atypical atrial flutter originating in the right atrial free wall. *Circulation*, 2000; **101**: 270–9.

40. Jais, P., D.C. Shah, M. Haissaguerre, *et al.* Mapping and ablation of left atrial flutters. *Circulation*, 2000; **101**: 2928–34.

41. Dorostkar, P.C., J. Cheng, M.M. Scheinman, Electroanatomical mapping and ablation of the substrate supporting intraatrial re-entrant tachycardia after palliation for complex congenital heart disease. *PACE*, 1998; **21**: 1810–19.

42. Leonelli, F.M., G. Tomassoni, M. Richey, A. Natale. Ablation of incisional atrial tachycardias using a three-dimensional nonfluoroscopic mapping system. *PACE*, 2001; **24**: 1653–9.

43. Nakagawa, H., N. Shah, K. Matsudaira, *et al.* Characterization of reentrant circuit in macroreentrant right atrial tachycardia after surgical repair of congenital heart disease. *Circulation*, 2001; **103**: 699–709.

44. Magnin-Poull, I., C. De Chillou, H. Miljoen, M. Andronache, E. Aliot. Mechanisms of right atrial tachycardia occurring late after surgical closure of atrial septal defects. *J. Cardiovasc. Electrophysiol.*, July 2005; **16**: 681–7.

45. Shah, D., P. Jais, A. Takahashi, *et al.* Dual-loop intra-atrial reentry in humans. *Circulation*, 2000; **101**: 631–9.

46. Marrouche, N.F., A. Natale, O.M. Wazni, *et al.* Left septal atrial flutter: electrophysiology, anatomy, and results of ablation. *Circulation*, 2004; **109**: 2440–7.

47. Reithmann, C., E. Hoffmann, U. Dorwarth, T. Remp, G. Steinbeck. Electroanatomical mapping for visualization of atrial activation in patients with incisional atrial tachycardias. *Eur. Heart J.*, 2001; **22**: 237–46.

48. Kantharia, B.K. Electroanatomical mapping and radiofrequency catheter ablation of atrial tachycardia originating from the recipient heart with recipient-to-donor atrio-atrial conduction after orthotopic heart transplantation. *J. Interv. Card. Electrophysiol.*, January 2005; **12**(1): 61–7.

49. Fuster, V., L.E. Ryden, D.S. Cannom, *et al.* ACC/AHA/ESC 2006 guidelines for the management of patients with atrial fibrillation: a report of the American College of Cardiology/American Heart Association Task Force on Practice Guidelines and the European Society of Cardiology Committee for Practice Guidelines. *Circulation*, 2006; **114**: 257–354.

50. Pappone, C., G. Oreto, F. Lamberti, *et al.* Catheter ablation of paroxysmal atrial fibrillation using 3D mapping system. *Circulation*, 1999; **100**: 1203–8.

51. Gepstein, L., T. Wolf, G. Hayam, S.A. Ben-Haim, Accurate linear radiofrequency lesions guided by a nonfluoroscopic electroanatomic mapping method during atrial fibrillation. *PACE*, 2001; **24**: 1672–8.

52. Ernst, S., M. Schluter, F. Ouyang, *et al.* Modification of the substrate for maintenance of idiopathic human atrial fibrillation: efficacy of radiofrequency ablation using nonfluoroscopic catheter guidance. *Circulation*, 1999; **100**: 2085–92.

53. Dong, J., H. Calkins, S.B. Solomon, *et al.* Integrated electroanatomic mapping with three-dimensional computed tomographic images for real-time guided ablations. *Circulation*, 2006; **113**: 186–94.

54. Kistler, P., K. Rajappan, M. Jahngir, *et al.* The impact of CT image integration into an electroanatomic mapping system on clinical outcomes of catheter ablation of atrial fibrillation. *J. Cardiovasc. Electrophysiol.*, October 2006; **17**: 1093–101.

55. Kistler, P.M., M.J. Earley, S. Harris, *et al.* Validation of three-dimensional cardiac image integration: use of integrated CT image into electroanatomic mapping system to perform catheter ablation of atrial fibrillation. *J. Cardiovasc. Electrophysiol.*, April 2006; **17**: 341–8.

56. Dong, J., T. Dickfeld, D. Dalal, *et al.* Initial experience in the use of integrated electroanatomic mapping with three-dimensional MR/CT images to guide catheter ablation of atrial fibrillation. *J. Cardiovasc. Electrophysiol.*, May 2006; **17**: 459–66.

57. Verma, A., O.M. Wazni, N.F. Marrouche, *et al.* Pre-existent left atrial scarring in patients undergoing pulmonary vein antrum isolation. *J. Am. Coll. Cardiol.*, 2005; **45**: 285–92.

58. Fahmy, T.S., H. Mlcochova, O.M. Wazni, *et al.* Intracardiac echo-guided image integration: optimizing strategies for registration. *J. Cardiovasc. Electrophysiol.*, 2007; **18**(3): 283–5.

59. Pappone, C., F. Manguso, G. Vicedomini, *et al.* Prevention of iatrogenic atrial tachycardia after ablation of atrial fibrillation. *Circulation*, 2004; **110**: 3036–42.

60. Jais P, M Hocini, LF Hsu, et al. Technique and results of linear ablation at the mitral isthmus. *Circulation*, 2004; **110**: 2996–3002.

61. Fassini G, S Riva, R Chiodelli et al. Left mitral isthmus ablation associated with PV isolation: long-term results of a prospective randomized study. *J. Cardiovasc. Electrophysiol.*, November 2005; **16**: 1150–6.

62. Duru F, G Hindricks, H Kottkamp. Atypical left atrial flutter after intraoperative radiofrequency ablation of chronic atrial fibrillation: successful ablation using

three-dimensional electroanatomic mapping. *J. Cardio-vasc. Electrophysiol.*, May 2001; **12**: 602–5.

63. Estner, H.L., I. Deisenhofer, A. Luik, *et al.* Electrical isolation of pulmonary veins in patients with atrial fibrillation: reduction of fluoroscopy exposure and procedure duration by the use of a non-fluoroscopic navigation system (NAVX). *Europace*, August 2006; **8**(8): 583–7.

64. Lang, C.C.E., F. Gugliotta, V. Santinelli, *et al.* Endocardial impedance mapping during circumferential pulmonary vein ablation of atrial fibrillation differentiates between atrial and venous tissue. *Heart Rhythm*, 2006; **3**: 171–8.

65. Piorkowski, C., G. Hindricks, D. Schreiber, *et al.* Electro-anatomic reconstruction of the left atrium, pulmonary veins, and esophagus compared with the "true anatomy" on multislice computed tomography in patients undergoing catheter ablation of atrial fibrillation. *Heart Rhythm*, 2006; **3**: 317–27.

66. Cummings, J.E., R.A. Schweikert, W.I. Saliba, *et al.* Assessment of temperature, proximity, and course of the esophagus during radiofrequency ablation within the left atrium. *Circulation*, 2005; **112**: 459–64.

67. Sherzer, A.I., D.Y. Feigenblum, S. Kulkarni, *et al.* Continuous nonfluoroscopic localization of the esophagus during radiofrequency catheter ablation of atrial fibrillation. *J. Cardiovasc. Electrophysiol.*, February 2007; **18**: 157–60.

68. Kim, Y-H., H-N. Pak, H.E. Lim, *et al.* Low voltage mapping and dominant frequency analysis of left atrial fibrillation. *Heart Rhythm*, 2006; Supp **3**(5): S328.

69. Jarman, J.W.E., T. Wong, H. Spohr, *et al.* Spectral analysis of atrial fibrillation using noncontact mapping to study the impact of circumferential ablation. *Heart Rhythm*, 2006; Supp **3**(5): S204.

CHAPTER 3

The utility of electroanatomical mapping in catheter ablation of ventricular tachycardias

Daejoon Anh, MD, *Henry H. Hsia*, MD, FACC, *& David J. Callans*, MD, FACC, FHRS

Introduction

The treatment of ventricular tachycardia (VT) has evolved significantly with the advent of catheter-based ablation. Successful VT ablation is critically dependent on accurate mapping of the arrhythmia to pinpoint the culprit tissue for destruction. The early pioneers in electrophysiology championed pace-mapping, activation-mapping, and entrainment-mapping techniques. Although these "conventional" mapping techniques have been further refined, they remain the cornerstones of even the most modern VT mapping strategy. Overreliance on the latest mapping technology without a basic understanding of anatomy, physiology, and careful attention to the electrogram recordings can often lead to unsuccessful outcomes. As an electroanatomic map is only as good as the information from which it is built from, the dictum "Garbage In, Garbage Out" should always be remembered when acquiring and interpreting the mapping data.

Nevertheless, the modern three-dimensional electroanatomic mapping technology is a powerful tool for mapping and ablation of VT, and in certain cases is critical in achieving desired outcomes. In particular, substrate-based ablation strategy for scar-based VT relies heavily on the three-dimensional mapping system to characterize the electroanatomical substrate and to delineate the potential areas for ablation.

Electroanatomical Mapping, 1st edition. Edited by
A. Al-Ahmad, D. Callans, H. Hsia and A. Natale.
© 2008 Blackwell Publishing, ISBN: 9781405157025.

The foremost utility of the three-dimensional mapping system is to provide a critical understanding of the spatial relationships between various cardiac structures. This coupled with the electrophysiologic data enables creation of a construct for the electroanatomical substrate. In this chapter, the applications of this technology in mapping focal idiopathic VT, reentrant VT utilizing the conduction system, and scar-based myocardial reentrant VTs will be discussed and illustrated.

Mapping of focal VT

Idiopathic VTs occurring in structurally normal hearts commonly arise from triggered activity or abnormal automaticity, and most often occur in perivalvular areas. These include VTs with site of origin at the mitral or tricuspid annulus [1,2], RV outflow tract (RVOT) [3], pulmonary artery [4], LV outflow tract (LVOT), or the aortic cusps [5,6]. In addition, idiopathic LV epicardial VTs occurring near the perivascular regions have already been described [7]. A 12-lead ECG of the VT offers substantive clues to the VT's site of origin and dictates which initial chamber is to be mapped [8]. At the same time, it should be recognized that some aspects of these structures are contiguous to each other, and consequently electrocardiographic distinction of cardiac chamber of origin may not always be accurate or possible.

The precise impact of electroanatomic mapping in ablation of idiopathic VT has not been studied in a prospective manner [9]. The utility of three-dimensional mapping technology provides the ability to display relative activation patterns across an anatomical region of interest and maintains a spatial log of points that produced promising pace-maps, allowing the operator to precisely "back-track" to the area of interest later in the procedure. Spatial resolution of less than 1 mm has been demonstrated with the CARTO™ electroanatomic mapping system, assuming reference position stability [10].

The VTs associated with structurally normal hearts most often have focal origin and are mapped predominantly with two methods: activation mapping and pace-mapping. Activation mapping searches for the earliest area of activation based on the local bipolar electrogram timing, and/or a QS pattern on unipolar recordings, as wave fronts propagate away from the focus. Relative timing of recorded signals can be assessed in reference to surface R waves or intracardiac ventricular electrograms (Figure 3.1). Activation isochronal maps can be constructed to display the area with the earliest isochronal time as an "early spot" (Figure 3.2).

However, the speed of wave front propagation from the site of origin to the adjacent tissue may be a factor in determining the accuracy of activation mapping, as areas with the earliest isochrone have been shown to be significantly larger in the presence of isoproterenol infusion [11]. In addition, local anisotropic conduction delay may also limit the value of unipolar recordings for activation mapping. An rS unipolar signal configuration can be observed as close as 2 mm from the site of origin, whereas a QS pattern may be recorded from a distant site [12].

Pace-mapping for localization of focal VT strives to reproduce the exact surface 12-lead QRS morphology with either unipolar or bipolar pacing at low-current outputs from a closely spaced bipole of a mapping catheter [13]. By providing localization information and tracking of catheter positions, electroanatomic mapping systems incorporate the pace-mapping results with anatomy and optimize the ability to achieve the best-matched QRS morphology. However, subtle variations in QRS morphology of the VT can be observed, which may be associated more than one distinct foci within a limited area [14,15]. Although previous studies have suggested that pace-mapping may be more precise in locating the site of origin compared with activation mapping for focal VTs, a more recent investigation has shown a comparable efficacy between pace-mapping and activation mapping with the magnetic electroanatomic mapping system [11].

In cases where the target VT or ventricular premature complexes (VPCs) are infrequently induced, the EnSite™ noncontact mapping system may be of value. Nonrandomized studies involving limited number of patients with RVOT VT or ventricular premature depolarizations (VPDs) have suggested potential benefits of this balloon-array-based noncontact mapping system that can record the global activation sequence in a single beat (Figure 3.3). Friedman *et al.* reported series of ten patients who underwent ablation for RVOT VT [16]. Acute success in nine patients and arrhythmia-free survival in seven patients in 11 months of follow-up was reported. Notably, seven of these patients have had previously unsuccessful ablations. Similarly, Ribbing *et al.* demonstrated 100% acute success in 12 patients undergoing ablations for RVOT VT or VPDs, and 11 of these patients remained arrhyth-

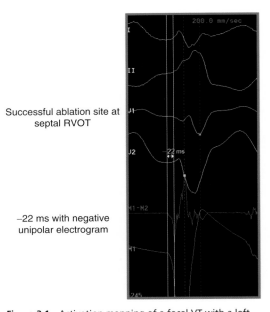

Successful ablation site at septal RVOT

−22 ms with negative unipolar electrogram

Figure 3.1 Activation mapping of a focal VT with a left-bundle-branch-block, inferior (LBBB-I) QRS axis, originating from the right ventricular outflow tract (RVOT). The unipolar electrogram (M1) recordings at the site of successful ablation demonstrated a "QS" configuration that was presystolic relative to the onset of surface QRS by 22 ms. The bipolar electrograms (M1–M2) had later activation timing than the unipolar recordings.

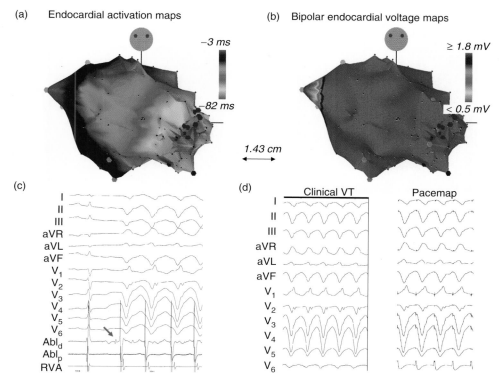

Figure 3.2 Endocardial three-dimensional electroanatomic mapping in a patient with monomorphic focal VT. (a) Activation map showed temporal isochronal color changes with the red colored area represents early activation (−82 ms) with late area is depicted by purple color (−3 ms). This represents centrifugal wave front propagation away from a focal early site (red spot). (b) Voltage map showed no evidence of low-voltage abnormal endocardium. Purple colored areas represent normal endocardium (amplitude ≥ 1.5 mV) with dense scar depicted as red (amplitude < 0.5 mV). The border zone (amplitude 0.5–1.5 mV) is defined as areas with the intermediate color gradient. (c) Activation mapping showed presystolic potentials (arrow) during tachycardia, and (d) showed pace-mapping with the paced QRS matched perfectly with that of the focal VT.

mia-free in 9 months of follow-up [14]. The authors reported that compared with historic controls undergoing ablations for RVOT with "conventional mapping approach" using activation and pace mapping, patients undergoing ablation with the noncontact mapping system had higher acute success rate (100% vs. 71.5%), but had higher number of RF applications (6.9 ± 2.2 vs. 4.2 ± 3.0) and longer procedure time (275.8 ± 70.4 min vs. 166.9 ± 34.3 min), and a longer but statistically nonsignificant fluoroscopy time.

Mapping of VT utilizing cardiac conduction system

The role of the His-Purkinje system (HPS) in the mechanisms of VT include the classic bundle branch macroreentry, interfascicular reentry, as well as VT where the circuit involves both the Purkinje fibers and myocardial scar [17,18]. In addition, focal VT arising from the Purkinje fibers with features consistent with automaticity, as well as polymorphic VT triggered by premature depolarization from the distal arborization of the HPS have also been reported [18–20].

Reentrant VT where the tachycardia circuit is dependent on the HPS can occur in patients with or without underlying structural heart disease [21–23]. Although bundle branch reentry (BBR) VT classically occurs in patients with nonischemic dilated cardiomyopathy and concomitant His-Purkinje conduction disease, this arrhythmia can occur in cardiomyopathies of any etiology [18,21,24–26]. Furthermore, in a heterogeneous group of patients with structural heart disease, 60% of the patients

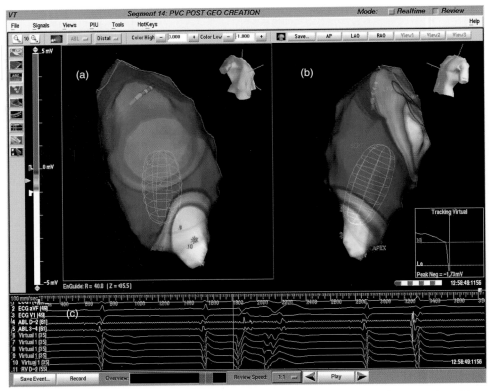

Figure 3.3 Single-beat activation mapping using the EnSite™ noncontact mapping system. The patient has a history of idiopathic left ventricular tachycardia and endocardial mapping was performed during isolated VPCs. Isochronal global activation maps were shown in right anterior oblique (RAO)-caudal (a) and left anterior oblique (LAO)-caudal (b) projections. The earliest site of activation was located at the apical inferior portion of the left ventricle (white zone). Six virtual unipolar electrogram recordings were displayed (c) and demonstrated a steep QS pattern with the earliest presystolic ventricular recording occurred at pole 10 (10 Virtual) that corresponds to the zone of early activation.

with BBR VT also have inducible for myocardial scar-based reentrant VT [18].

As patients with cardiomyopathy and underlying myocardial scar may have the substrates for both HPS-mediated VT and scar-based reentrant VT, it is important to make the diagnostic distinction as the ablative strategies differ substantially [18]. The diagnosis of BBR VT is first suggested by characteristic surface ECG morphologies. The QRS morphology during VT often bears similarity to that of sinus rhythm QRS with a typical left bundle branch block (LBBB) or right bundle branch block (RBBB) appearance. The diagnosis is confirmed by careful electrogram recordings of the HPS potentials during VT. Involvement of the HPS in this circus movement reentry can also be established by entrainment from either the right bundle branch

or the left fascicle [17,18,27]. Locations of the bundle branches can be easily defined and displayed on three-dimensional electroanatomic maps and catheter ablation of the right or left bundle branches interrupts the circuit and provides an effective treatment of this arrhythmia.

The mechanism of idiopathic left ventricular VT (Belhassen VT), typically involves reentry using the left-sided fascicles-Purkinje network [28]. The reentry commonly depends on verapamil-sensitive tissue with slow conduction and an excitable gap, [23,29]. Although such "verapamil-sensitive VT" has been traditionally thought to occur exclusively in patients with structurally normal hearts, reentrant monomorphic VT originating from the left posterior Purkinje fibers has also been reported in patients with postinfarction cardiomyopathy [27].

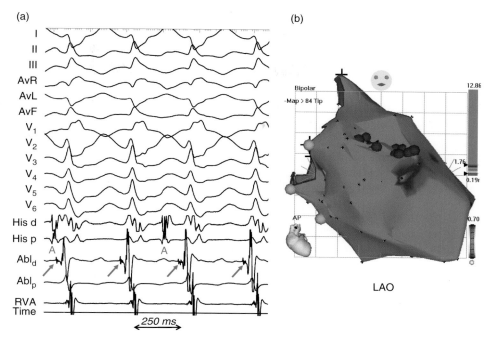

Figure 3.4 Empiric linear ablations of the left anterior fascicle in a patient with fascicular tachycardia. Presystolic Purkinje potentials were noted (arrows) during a right bundle branch block, right inferior (RBRI) QRS VT (a). The left ventricular voltage map showed no evidence of endocardial scar and the color gradient corresponds to the left ventricular electrogram amplitude as described in Figure 3.2. Ablation line transacting the left anterior fascicle successfully eliminated the tachycardia (b).

In addition, scar-related reentrant VT where the exit occurs through the posterior Purkinje fibers may also mimic the Belhassen VT [17].

Components of the HPS can be mapped during sinus rhythm by looking for sharp, high-frequency potentials. Such "substrate map" of the HPS can be created by tagging the potential locations. The utility of electroanatomic mapping in catheter ablation of His-Purkinje-mediated VTs was highlighted by Ouyang *et al.* [23]. In this study, electroanatomical mapping of the left fascicular conduction system was performed in patients with left posterior fascicular VTs during sinus rhythm. Importantly, all patients with fascicular VT demonstrated sites with late-systolic Purkinje potentials (PP) in addition to a presystolic PP during sinus rhythm, whereas the control patients only demonstrated presystolic PP. The late-systolic PPs in sinus rhythm appear to represent retrograde wave front invasion into the Purkinje network with conduction delay, which constitute the substrate for reentry within the fascicular system. Indeed, sites with the late-systolic retrograde Purkinje potentials in sinus rhythm were proven to be part of the reentrant circuit by entrainment mapping and were successfully targeted for ablation. The ability to mark the location of the HPS during sinus rhythm by electroanatomic mapping not only facilitate the ability to accurately return to these areas to perform additional mapping maneuvers, but also allows empiric ablations of the putative circuit involving the HPS, particularly if the VT is nonsustained or noninducible. Notably, ablation at the earliest retrograde PP in sinus rhythm was also successful in controlling the VT in clinical follow-up. Others have reported successful outcomes with similar empiric ablation strategies utilizing an electroanatomic His-Purkinje "substrate map" (Figure 3.4) [30]. Thus, it appears that the ability to map and record a sequence of Purkinje potentials on the three-dimensional map offers distinct advantages in successful ablative outcome in fascicular VT.

Recently, polymorphic VT/ ventricular fibrillation (VF) triggered by ventricular premature complexes (VPCs) after a myocardial infarction have been reported [19,20,31]. Szumowski *et al.* found that all "triggered" VPCs were mapped to the Purkinje network near the myocardial infarction, within 1 cm of the myocardial scar as defined by electroanatomic voltage map. These culprit ventricular premature beats appear to originate from the surviving Purkinje fibers at the border zone of infarction and were always preceded by a Purkinje potential at the site of earliest activation [20]. Mapping and ablation of these abnormal Purkinje fibers have been shown to prevent recurrent ventricular tachyarrhythmias. Moreover, empiric ablation of Purkinje potentials within the border zone of infarction in patients who were not inducible for triggering ventricular beats led to effective treatment of VT/VF [31].

Mapping of scar-based reentrant VT

Much of what is known about ventricular arrhythmias is based on studies of ischemic heart disease. Results of surgical mapping studies indicate that reentrant ventricular tachycardias often originate from subendocardial sites of infarcted myocardium adjacent to the densely scarred aneurysm [32–34]. Surviving endocardial myocardial fibers surrounded by extensive fibrosis form the basis of slow and nonuniform anisotropic conductive channels that can act as the critical isthmus of the VT. The amplitude of the abnormal endocardial electrogram is related to the number of viable muscle fibers under the recording electrode, whereas the degree of electrogram fractionation is associated with the extent of electrical decoupling and anisotropy [35]. Consequently, the electrophysiological substrate of potential VT circuits is often manifested by the presence of low-amplitude, prolonged, and fractionated electrogram signals.

As such, identification and characterization of the myocardial scar that constitutes the substrate for reentrant VT plays a critical role in successful ablation outcome. Kornowski *et al.* were the first to demonstrate the feasibility of magnetic electroanatomic mapping technique in distinguishing infarcted myocardium from healthy tissue [36]. The accuracy of electroanatomic mapping in determining infarct scar size and location in a porcine model

was analyzed by different investigators [37,38]. The endocardial area bounded by contiguous abnormal bipolar electrogram recordings with bipolar signal amplitudes less than 1 mV correlated well with pathologic analysis. In addition, the area of akinesis determined by intracardiac echocardiography correlated well with the area of contiguous abnormal electrogram distribution with a bipolar signal of amplitude less than 2 mV. The infarct location and border zone geometry were also accurately described by the three-dimensional electroanatomic voltage mapping. These findings have also been confirmed by limited pathologic analysis in humans, where the local bipolar electrogram voltage has been correlated to the degree of tissue scarring/fibrosis [39,40].

The normal reference range of electrogram amplitude for electroanatomic mapping using the Biosense-CARTO™ system (Biosense Webster, Inc.) has been studied in humans by Marchlinski *et al.* [41]. The mean bipolar electrogram amplitude in the normal LV endocardium obtained during sinus rhythm was 4.8 ± 3.1 mV, where 95% of all LV electrograms were greater than 1.55 mV. Similarly, the mean bipolar electrogram amplitude recorded from the normal right ventricle was 3.7 ± 1.7 mV, with 95% of all electrogram recordings being greater than 1.44 mV. Based on these data, a bipolar electrogram amplitude (voltage) greater than 1.5 mV is defined as "normal" endocardium (<20% fibrosis). It is noteworthy that reference values for normal endocardial electrogram amplitude have not been established for other mapping systems.

Although abnormal electrogram amplitude for ventricles is widely accepted as less than 1.5 mV, densely "scarred" endocardium has been *arbitrarily* defined as less than 0.5 mV based on prior surgical experiences. Tissues with local bipolar voltage between 0.5 and 1.5 mV is considered in the abnormal "border zone", commonly adjacent to the dense scar and normal myocardium. Tissues with local bipolar electrogram voltage less than 0.5 mV have been correlated to extensive underlying fibrosis involving more than 80% of the volume, while the border zone (0.5–1.5 mV) corresponds to an intermediate degree (20–80%) of scarring [39].

The anatomy of the endocardial substrate of ventricular tachycardia was recently characterized in a heterogeneous group of patients with structural

Table 3.1 Correlation of local electrogram amplitude profile and the reentrant VT circuit.

	Entrance	Central isthmus	Exit	Outer loop
Dense scar (<0.5 mV)	17	30	18	6
Border zone (0.5–1.5 mV)	2	7	26	18
Normal (>1.5 mV)	–	–	4	8
Total	19	37	48	32

heart disease who presented with uniform VT [42]. Detailed entrainment mapping was performed during all hemodynamically stable sustained monomorphic VTs and the endocardial dimension and local electrogram voltage profile of the reentry circuits was determined. Eighty-four percent of the entrance or isthmus sites were located within "dense scar" (<0.5 mV), while nearly all exits (92%) were located in abnormal endocardium (<1.5 mV) with over half (54%) located in border zone (0.5–1.5 mV) (Table 3.1). Other investigators have also identified the VT exit at or near the border zone that can be successfully targeted for ablation [43]. The endocardial extent of the VT circuit was highly variable and generally involves a distance of at least several centimeters in length (average 35±23 mm).

Some investigators have found a bipolar signal amplitude threshold of <0.05 or <0.1 mV to be a more useful cutoff point to define dense scar [41,44–46]. Indeed, an alternative definition of a "true" dense scar is by its electrical inexcitability, and the local capture threshold has shown to be inversely correlated with the recorded electrogram amplitude. Electrical unexcitable scar (EUS) has been identified by noncapture with high-output unipolar pacing (>10 mA). Such dense scar tissue has shown to be commonly in proximity to the zone of slow conduction (isthmus) of the VT circuit and may help to define the boundaries of the conducting channels (Figure 3.5) [47]. Caution is needed when substrate mapping the epicardial surface as fibrofatty tissue overlying normal myocardium can be interpreted as a low-voltage scarred area [40,48].

Surviving myofibers within the zone of slow conduction are often located within the abnormal myocardium and adjacent to dense scar [49]. Electrogram recordings from these areas may exhibit a higher signal amplitude/voltage compared with the surrounding nonconducting scar. The presence of

such viable myocardium within areas of low-voltage scar represents a potential conducting channel can now be identified using high-density electroanatomical mapping (Figure 3.6). A conducting channel is defined as a path demonstrating contiguous electrograms with voltage higher than that of the surrounding areas as evidenced by distinct color differences with voltage threshold adjustment [42,50]. By carefully adjusting both the upper and lower voltage thresholds on the CARTO™ voltage map, a "corridor" demonstrating higher voltage amplitude than that of the surrounding areas could be visualized [42,50]. Notably, a single voltage threshold cutoff may not be feasible in all cases. In addition, complete and incomplete channels can be visualized that may not be related to the clinical VT. The relationship of such "conducting channels" to clinical VT circuits can often be confirmed by (1) concealed entrainment by pacing from within the channel; (2) local capture with perfect pace-mapping and a long stimulus-QRS interval; (3) activation mapping with early presystolic potentials; and (4) local electrograms with multiple fractionated/delayed component recorded within the channels [17,42,50]. RF ablation targeting tissues within the channels have also been shown to be effective in suppressing VT inducibility [42,50].

The optimal scar voltage definition for identification of most channels has been shown to be approximately 0.2–0.3 mV with a wide range (0.1–0.7 mV) [42,50]. These data are closely concordant with other studies for characterization of the VT isthmus using various methods (Table 3.2) [45,47,51].

In addition of defining the pathologic substrate, electroanatomic mapping may provide diagnostic information and risk stratification, particularly in patients with arrhythmogenic right ventricular dysplasia (ARVD). Sinus rhythm electroanatomic map of the right ventricle using CARTO™ in patients

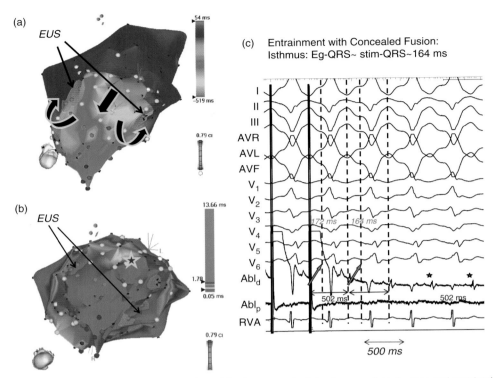

Figure 3.5 Electroanatomical mapping in a patient with a large anterior-lateral myocardial infarction and sustained monomorphic ventricular tachycardia. (a) Activation mapping during VT showed a "figure-of-eight" reentry. Temporal isochronal color changes demonstrated an "early-meets-late" activation pattern with the red color represents early activation and late area was depicted by purple color. Electrical unexcitable scar (EUS) was identified by noncapture with high-output pacing and is depicted by the gray scar (arrows). Such dense scar tissues commonly are in proximity to the zone of slow conduction/isthmus of the VT circuit and are often located deep in low voltage (<0.5 mV) area. (b) Voltage map showed a large anterior lateral scar with its borders defined by EUS. VT-related conducting channel is located between EUS and deep in the scar, and pacing (star) adjacent to EUS resulted in entrainment with concealed fusion.

with a clinical diagnosis of ARVD often demonstrates low-amplitude, fractionated electrograms with prolonged duration that is anatomically concordant with dyskinetic regions seen with imaging. In addition, fibrofatty infiltration and loss of myocytes seen on endomyocardial biopsy are associated with abnormal electroanatomic maps [52,53]. On the other hand, patients with clinical diagnosis of ARVD and a normal electroanatomic map of the right ventricle most often show histopathologic evidence of inflammatory cardiomyopathy. Notably, a normal right ventricular electroanatomic map is associated with a significantly better clinical outcome, even in patients who fulfil the diagnostic criteria set by the international study group for ARVD [52]. Therefore, electroanatomic substrate

mapping of the right ventricle can identify the underlying myopathic process in ARVD and may play an important role in risk stratification.

Although individual electrogram characteristic and/or amplitude may change with different activation sequences, the local bipolar amplitude has been shown to be closely correlated irrespective of the underlying rhythm (atrial pacing vs. right ventricular pacing) [54]. Based on our previous observations, voltage maps constructed during sinus rhythm and sustained monomorphic VT showed similar locations of abnormal endocardium with nearly identical distribution of "dense scar" and "border zone" (Figure 3.7) [42]. With high-density mapping, the overall distribution of electrogram pattern should not be significantly affected, and

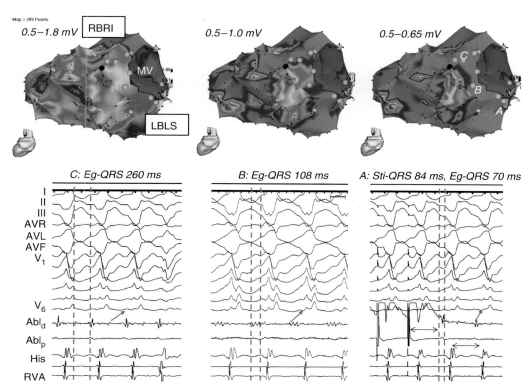

Figure 3.6 Identification of VT-related conducting channel in a patient with prior myocardial infarctions who presented with sustained VT. Two tachycardias were documented with a right bundle branch block, right inferior (RBRI) and a left bundle branch block, left superior (LBLS) QRS morphologies. By carefully adjusting the upper and lower color voltage thresholds on the electroanatomic voltage map (0.5–1.8 mV, 0.5–1.0 mV, and 0.5–0.65 mV), a corridor demonstrating higher voltage amplitude than that of the surrounding areas could be visualized. Entrainment with concealed fusion within the channel was noted at multiple sites (A, B, and C) with progressively longer stimulus-QRS (Sti-QRS) intervals that equaled electrogram-QRS (Eg-QRS) intervals. This is an example of mitral annular VT with counterclockwise (LBLS) and clockwise reentry (RBRI) VTs around the mitral valve.

Table 3.2 Comparisons of isthmus characteristics of reentrant VT circuits.

References	Mapping techniques	Isthmus length (mm)	Voltage (mV)	Mapping features
Soejima et al. (2002)	Pace-mapping entrainment	26 ± 14	0.32 ± 0.16 (0.08–0.91)	Near EUS
de Chillou et al. (2002)	Activation mapping, anatomic	31 ± 7	None	Diastolic and double potentials
Arenal et al. (2004)	Activation, pace-mapping, entrainment	23 ± 11	0.1–0.5 (~0.2)	E-IDC channels
Hsia et al. (2006)	Entrainment	31 ± 21	0.33 ± 0.15	Channels
Brunckhorst et al. (2004)	Pace-mapping entrainment	24 ± 6	< 1.5	S-QRS > 40 ms

EUS: Electrical unexcitable scar; E-IDC: Electrograms with isolated delayed components.

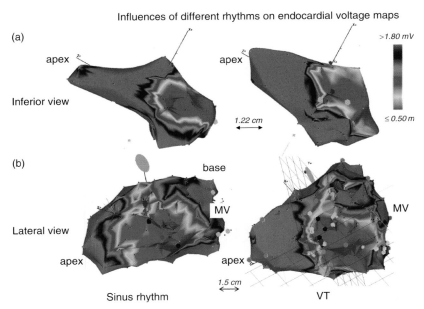

Influences of different rhythms on endocardial voltage maps

(a) Inferior view — apex ... apex, 1.22 cm, >1.80 mV, ≤0.50 m

(b) Lateral view — base, MV, MV, apex, apex, 1.5 cm

Sinus rhythm   VT

Figure 3.7 The influences of different rhythms on endocardial voltage maps. The color gradient corresponds to the left ventricular electrogram amplitude as described in Figure 3.2. Electroanatomic voltage maps were constructed during sinus rhythm and sustained monomorphic VT that showed similar locations of abnormal endocardium with nearly identical distribution of "dense scar" and "border zone".

electroanatomical maps accurately reflect the underlying voltage distribution regardless of the underlying rhythm.

Limitations

Electroanatomic mapping is an effective tool in delineating the underlying anatomy and pathology responsible for ventricular tachycardia. Although computerized construct is extremely valuable for the understanding of complex arrhythmias and anatomy, these maps require careful interpretation and knowledge of physiology. Overreliance without an understanding of its limitations often results in unfavorable outcomes.

Where it may fail most often relates to the poor signal quality of electrogram recordings and insufficient sampling frequency. Acquiring data points without ensuring good catheter contact and stability can give rise to apparent areas of abnormal low-voltage myocardium which may be misinterpreted as scar (Figure 3.8). Low number of sampling with fewer electrogram recordings often results in an inadequate characterization of the underlying anatomy, as well as an insufficient

display of the activation isochrones for activation mapping. Overrepresentation or underdetection of abnormal myocardium can also occur with a lack of adequate corroborative voltage data.

Severe derangement of activation maps can result from acquiring far-field, rather than local, electrograms during data collection. Moreover, selecting the amplitude of a nonlocal electrogram signal can erroneously represent the pattern of distribution of abnormal myocardium for substrate mapping. Lastly, the presence of endocardial thrombus or epicardial fat can easily mimic a "scar" on a voltage map [48].

Conclusions

Electroanatomic mapping is an important and essential component for successful mapping and ablation of a diverse population of ventricular tachycardias. High-density three-dimensional electroanatomical mapping provides detailed spatial relationships between various cardiac structures, as well as characterization of the arrhythmogenic substrate. It is essential in the paradigm of "substrate-based mapping", particularly for VTs that are

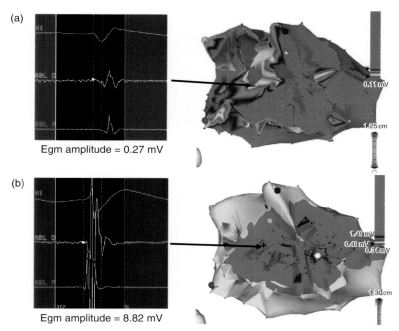

Egm amplitude = 0.27 mV

Egm amplitude = 8.82 mV

Figure 3.8 The effect of catheter contact on electrogram voltage recordings and scar definition. Endocardial left ventricular electroanatomic mapping was performed in a patient with nonischemic cardiomyopathy with monomorphic VT. The color gradient corresponds to the left ventricular endocardial bipolar electrogram amplitude as described in Figure 3.1. The initial voltage map (a) demonstrated an area of abnormally low electrogram amplitude (<0.5 mV), consistent with a posterior septal scar in the right anterior oblique projection. Left panel showed local bipolar electrograms (Egm) with a wide signal width, slow slew rate and low signal amplitude measured at 0.27 mV. Note the "sunken-in" appearance of the anatomical shell, suggesting possible points with poor electrode-to-tissue contact. The electroanatomic map was further augmented by repeated high-density sampling over an existing "shell" (grey color). Good catheter contact for optimal recordings was carefully attended to. The resulting map (b) clearly demonstrated normal endocardial voltages in the posterior septum without evidence of scar. The local bipolar electrogram recordings showed large signal amplitude (8.82 mV) with a fast slew rate over the same location.

not amendable to the conventional mapping techniques. Various strategies may be used to identify and localize the putative circuit in scar-based reentry. These include (1) abnormal low local bipolar electrogram voltage/amplitude; (2) the presence of VT-related conducting channels (CC); (3) presence of dense scar as defined by electrical inexcitability; (4) identification and localization of electrogram recordings with isolated delayed components; and (5) pace mapping to define zone of slow conduction with long stimulus-QRS intervals.

What is the best approach for catheter ablation of VT? A single mapping method may not be suitable for all VTs (both mappable and unmappable). An integrated approach using a "tailored" substrate mapping with a combination of voltage analysis, activation mapping, together with the identification of conduction channels and EUS, as well as

targeting areas of interest with fractionated and/or late potentials may result in the most accurate, efficient, and successful outcome [17,55,56]. The contribution of pace mapping to the identification of candidate sites for RF ablation remains important. Limited activation mapping or entrainment mapping of VT at preselected sites is useful for confirming the target location. The design of RF ablation lines must be tailored to the degree of reliability and precision of the mapping data. Placement of ablation lines designed to transect the preferred conduction channels in abnormal scar and border zone regions may facilitate ablation of multiple stable and unstable VTs, even in the absence of VT induction.

Although substrate mapping of the ventricle is important in scar-related VT, it is also a time-consuming process and many patients with ventricular tachycardia may not be able to tolerate prolonged procedures. High-density mapping of a limited area guided by limited pace-mapping and entrainment mapping can shorten the procedural time without significantly compromising outcomes [57]. Promising advances in robotic and magnetic catheter manipulation and incorporation of other imaging modalities such as computed tomography or ultrasound into the electroanatomic mapping process may enhance the ability of the electrophysiologist to efficiently map and ablate ventricular tachycardias in the future.

References

1. Tada, H., S. Ito, S. Naito, *et al.*, Idiopathic ventricular arrhythmia arising from the mitral annulus: a distinct subgroup of idiopathic ventricular arrhythmias. *J. Am. Coll. Cardiol.*, 2005; **45**: 877–86.
2. Tada, H., K. Tadokoro, S. Ito, *et al.*, Idiopathic ventricular arrhythmias originating from the tricuspid annulus: prevalence, electrocardiographic characteristics, and results of radiofrequency catheter ablation. *Heart Rhythm*, 2007; **4**: 7–16.
3. Morady, F., A.H. Kadish, L. DiCarlo, *et al.*, Long-term results of catheter ablation of idiopathic right ventricular tachycardia. *Circulation*, 1990; **82**: 2093–9.
4. Timmermans, C., L.M. Rodriguez, H.J. Crijns, A.F. Moorman, and H.J. Wellens, Idiopathic left bundle-branch block-shaped ventricular tachycardia may originate above the pulmonary valve. *Circulation*, 2003; **108**: 1960–7.
5. Schweikert, R.A., W.I. Saliba, G. Tomassoni, *et al.*, Percutaneous pericardial instrumentation for endo-epicardial mapping of previously failed ablations. *Circulation*, 2003; **108**: 1329–35.
6. Ouyang, F., P. Fotuhi, S.Y. Ho, *et al.*, Repetitive monomorphic ventricular tachycardia originating from the aortic sinus cusp: electrocardiographic characterization for guiding catheter ablation. *J. Am. Coll. Cardiol.*, 2002; **39**: 500–8.
7. Daniels, D.V., Y.Y. Lu, J.B. Morton, *et al.*, Idiopathic epicardial left ventricular tachycardia originating remote from the sinus of Valsalva: electrophysiological characteristics, catheter ablation, and identification from the 12-lead electrocardiogram. *Circulation*, 2006; **113**: 1659–66.
8. Badhwar, N. and M.M. Scheinman, Idiopathic ventricular tachycardia: diagnosis and management. *Curr. Probl. Cardiol.*, 2007; **32**: 7–43.
9. Saleem, M.A., S. Burkett, R. Passman, *et al.*, New simplified technique for 3D mapping and ablation of right ventricular outflow tract tachycardia. *Pacing Clin. Electrophysiol.*, 2005; **28**: 397–403.
10. Gepstein, L., G. Hayam, and S.A. Ben-Haim, A novel method for nonfluoroscopic catheter-based electroanatomical mapping of the heart: *in vitro* and *in vivo* accuracy results. In; 1997; 1611–22.
11. Azegami, K., D.J. Wilber, M. Arruda, A.C. Lin, and R.A. Denman, Spatial resolution of pacemapping and activation mapping in patients with idiopathic right ventricular outflow tract tachycardia. *J. Cardiovasc. Electrophysiol.*, 2005; **16**: 823–9.
12. Man, K.C., E.G. Daoud, B.P. Knight, *et al.*, Accuracy of the unipolar electrogram for identification of the site of origin of ventricular activation. *J. Cardiovasc. Electrophysiol.*, 1997; **8**: 974–9.
13. Kadish, A.H., S. Schmaltz, and F. Morady, A comparison of QRS complexes resulting from unipolar and bipolar pacing: implications for pace-mapping. *Pacing Clin. Electrophysiol.*, 1991; **14**: 823–32.
14. Ribbing, M., K. Wasmer, G. Monnig, *et al.*, Endocardial mapping of right ventricular outflow tract tachycardia using noncontact activation mapping. *J. Cardiovasc. Electrophysiol.*, 2003; **14**: 602–8.
15. Chinushi, M., Y. Aizawa, K. Takahashi, H. Kitazawa, and A. Shibata, Radiofrequency catheter ablation for idiopathic right ventricular tachycardia with special reference to morphological variation and long-term outcome. *Heart*, 1997; **78**: 255–61.
16. Friedman, P.A., S.J. Asirvatham, S. Grice, *et al.*, Noncontact mapping to guide ablation of right ventricular outflow tract tachycardia. *J. Am. Coll. Cardiol.*, 2002; **39**: 1808–12.
17. Bogun, F., E. Good, S. Reich, *et al.*, Role of Purkinje fibers in post-infarction ventricular tachycardia. *J. Am. Coll. Cardiol.*, 2006; **48**: 2500–7.
18. Lopera, G., W.G. Stevenson, K. Soejima, *et al.*, Identification and ablation of three types of ventricular tachycardia involving the His-Purkinje system in patients with heart disease. *J. Cardiovasc. Electrophysiol.*, 2004; **15**: 52–8.
19. Bansch, D., F. Oyang, M. Antz, *et al.*, Successful catheter ablation of electrical storm after myocardial infarction. *Circulation*, 2003; **108**: 3011–16.
20. Szumowski, L., P. Sanders, F. Walczak, *et al.*, Mapping and ablation of polymorphic ventricular tachycardia after myocardial infarction. *J. Am. Coll. Cardiol.*, 2004; **44**: 1700–6.
21. Hsia, H.H. and F.E. Marchlinski, Characterization of the electroanatomic substrate for monomorphic ventricular tachycardia in patients with nonischemic cardiomyopathy. *Pacing Clin. Electrophysiol.*, 2002; **25**: 1114–27.
22. Merino, J.L., R. Peinado, I. Fernandez-Lozano, N. Sobrino, and J.A. Sobrino, Transient entrainment of bundle-branch reentry by atrial and ventricular stimulation: elucidation of the tachycardia mechanism through analysis of the surface ECG. *Circulation*, 1999; **100**: 1784–90.

23. Ouyang, F., R. Cappato, S. Ernst, *et al.*, Electroanatomic substrate of idiopathic left ventricular tachycardia: unidirectional block and macroreentry within the purkinje network. *Circulation*, 2002; **105**: 462–9.

24. Akhtar, M., S. Denker, M.H. Lehmann, and R. Mahmud, Macro-reentry within the His Purkinje system. *Pacing Clin. Electrophysiol.*, 1983; **6**: 1010–28.

25. Caceres, J., M. Jazayeri, J. McKinnie, *et al.*, Sustained bundle branch reentry as a mechanism of clinical tachycardia. *Circulation*, 1989; **79**: 256–70.

26. Blanck, Z., S. Deshpande, M.R. Jazayeri, and M. Akhtar, Catheter ablation of the left bundle branch for the treatment of sustained bundle branch reentrant ventricular tachycardia. *J. Cardiovasc. Electrophysiol.*, 1995; **6**: 40–3.

27. Hayashi, M., Y. Kobayashi, Y.K. Iwasaki, *et al.*, Novel mechanism of postinfarction ventricular tachycardia originating in surviving left posterior Purkinje fibers. *Heart Rhythm*, 2006; **3**: 908–18.

28. Belhassen, B., I. Shapira, A. Pelleg, I. Copperman, N. Kauli, and S. Laniado, Idiopathic recurrent sustained ventricular tachycardia responsive to verapamil: an ECG-electrophysiologic entity. *Am. Heart J.*, 1984; **108**: 1034–7.

29. Sethi, K., B. Singh, G. Kalra, *et al.*, Verapamil responsive ventricular tachycardia: clinical and electrophysiologic characteristics. *Indian Heart J.*, 1991; **43**: 437–43.

30. Lin, D., H.H. Hsia, E.P. Gerstenfeld, *et al.*, Idiopathic fascicular left ventricular tachycardia: linear ablation lesion strategy for noninducible or nonsustained tachycardia. *Heart Rhythm*, 2005; **2**: 934–9.

31. Marrouche, N.F., A. Verma, O. Wazni, *et al.*, Mode of initiation and ablation of ventricular fibrillation storms in patients with ischemic cardiomyopathy. *J. Am. Coll. Cardiol.*, 2004; **43**: 1715–20.

32. Josephson, M.E., L.N. Horowitz, A. Farshidi, J.F. Spear, J.A. Kastor, and E.N. Moore, Recurrent sustained ventricular tachycardia. 2. Endocardial mapping. *Circulation*, 1978; **57**: 440–7.

33. Josephson, M.E., L.N. Horowitz, S.R. Spielman, A.M. Greenspan, C. VandePol, and A.H. Harken, Comparison of endocardial catheter mapping with intraoperative mapping of ventricular tachycardia. *Circulation*, 1980; **61**: 395–404.

34. Fenoglio, J.J., Jr., T.D. Pham, A.H. Harken, L.N. Horowitz, M.E. Josephson, and A.L. Wit, Recurrent sustained ventricular tachycardia: structure and ultrastructure of subendocardial regions in which tachycardia originates. *Circulation*, 1983; **68**: 518–33.

35. Gardner, P.I., P.C. Ursell, J.J. Fenoglio, Jr., and A.L. Wit, Electrophysiologic and anatomic basis for fractionated electrograms recorded from healed myocardial infarcts. *Circulation*, 1985; **72**: 596–611.

36. Kornowski, R., M.K. Hong, L. Gepstein, *et al.*, Preliminary animal and clinical experiences using an electromechanical endocardial mapping procedure to distinguish infarcted from healthy myocardium. *Circulation*, 1998; **98**: 1116–24.

37. Callans, D.J., J.F. Ren, J. Michele, F.E. Marchlinski, and S.M. Dillon, Electroanatomic left ventricular mapping in the porcine model of healed anterior myocardial infarction. Correlation with intracardiac echocardiography and pathological analysis. *Circulation*, 1999; **100**: 1744–50.

38. Wrobleski, D., C. Houghtaling, M.E. Josephson, J.N. Ruskin, and V.Y. Reddy, Use of electrogram characteristics during sinus rhythm to delineate the endocardial scar in a porcine model of healed myocardial infarction. *J. Cardiovasc. Electrophysiol.*, 2003; **14**: 524–9.

39. Deneke, T., K.M. Muller, B. Lemke, *et al.*, Human histopathology of electroanatomic mapping after cooled-tip radiofrequency ablation to treat ventricular tachycardia in remote myocardial infarction. *J. Cardiovasc. Electrophysiol.*, 2005; **16**: 1246–51.

40. Cesario, D.A., M. Vaseghi, N.G. Boyle, *et al.*, Value of high-density endocardial and epicardial mapping for catheter ablation of hemodynamically unstable ventricular tachycardia. *Heart Rhythm*, 2006; **3**: 1–10.

41. Marchlinski, F.E., D.J. Callans, C.D. Gottlieb, and E. Zado, Linear ablation lesions for control of unmappable ventricular tachycardia in patients with ischemic and nonischemic cardiomyopathy. *Circulation*, 2000; **101**: 1288–96.

42. Hsia, H.H., D. Lin, W.H. Sauer, D.J. Callans, and F.E. Marchlinski, Anatomic characterization of endocardial substrate for hemodynamically stable reentrant ventricular tachycardia: identification of endocardial conducting channels. *Heart Rhythm*, 2006; **3**: 503–12.

43. Verma, A., F. Kilicaslan, R.A. Schweikert, *et al.*, Short- and long-term success of substrate-based mapping and ablation of ventricular tachycardia in arrhythmogenic right ventricular dysplasia. *Circulation*, 2005; **111**: 3209–16.

44. Soejima, K., W.G. Stevenson, J.L. Sapp, A.P. Selwyn, G. Couper, and L.M. Epstein, Endocardial and epicardial radiofrequency ablation of ventricular tachycardia associated with dilated cardiomyopathy: the importance of low-voltage scars. *J. Am. Coll. Cardiol.*, 2004; **43**: 1834–42.

45. de Chillou, C., D. Lacroix, D. Klug, *et al.*, Isthmus characteristics of reentrant ventricular tachycardia after myocardial infarction. *Circulation*, 2002; **105**: 726–31.

46. Josephson, M.E., Electrophysiology of ventricular tachycardia: a historical perspective. *Pacing Clin. Electrophysiol.*, 2003; **26**: 2052–67.

47. Soejima, K., W.G. Stevenson, W.H. Maisel, J.L. Sapp, and L.M. Epstein, Electrically unexcitable scar mapping based on pacing threshold for identification of the

reentry circuit isthmus: feasibility for guiding ventricular tachycardia ablation. *Circulation*, 2002; **106**: 1678–83.

48. Dixit, S., N. Narula, D.J. Callans, and F.E. Marchlinski, Electroanatomic mapping of human heart: epicardial fat can mimic scar. *J. Cardiovasc. Electrophysiol.*, 2003; **14**: 1128.

49. de Bakker, J.M., F.J. van Capelle, M.J. Janse, *et al.*, Slow conduction in the infarcted human heart. 'Zigzag' course of activation. *Circulation*, 1993; **88**: 915–26.

50. Arenal, A., S. del Castillo, E. Gonzalez-Torrecilla, *et al.*, Tachycardia-related channel in the scar tissue in patients with sustained monomorphic ventricular tachycardias: influence of the voltage scar definition. *Circulation*, 2004; **110**: 2568–74.

51. Brunckhorst, C.B., E. Delacretaz, K. Soejima, W.H. Maisel, P.L. Friedman, and W.G. Stevenson, Identification of the ventricular tachycardia isthmus after infarction by pace mapping. *Circulation*, 2004; **110**: 652–9.

52. Corrado, D., C. Basso, L. Leoni, *et al.*, Three-dimensional electroanatomic voltage mapping increases accuracy of diagnosing arrhythmogenic right ventricular cardiomyopathy/dysplasia. *Circulation*, 2005; **111**: 3042–50.

53. Boulos, M., I. Lashevsky, and L. Gepstein, Usefulness of electroanatomical mapping to differentiate between right ventricular outflow tract tachycardia and arrhythmogenic right ventricular dysplasia. *Am. J. Cardiol.*, 2005; **95**: 935–40.

54. Brunckhorst, C., E. Delacretaz, K. Soejima, W. Maisel, P. Friedman, and W. Stevenson, Impact of changing activation sequence on bipolar electrogram amplitude for voltage mapping of left ventricular infarcts causing ventricular tachycardia. *J. Interv. Card. Electrophysiol.*, 2005; **12**: 137–41.

55. Hsia, H.H., Substrate mapping: the historical perspective and current status. *J. Cardiovasc. Electrophysiol.*, 2003; **14**: 530–2.

56. Delacretaz, E. and W.G. Stevenson, Catheter ablation of ventricular tachycardia in patients with coronary heart disease: part I: mapping. *Pacing Clin. Electrophysiol.*, 2001; **24**: 1261–77.

57. Kottkamp, H., U. Wetzel, P. Schirdewahn, *et al.*, Catheter ablation of ventricular tachycardia in remote myocardial infarction: substrate description guiding placement of individual linear lesions targetting noninducibility. *J. Cardiovasc. Electrophysiol.*, 2003; **14**: 675–81.

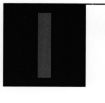

PART I

SVT cases

CHAPTER 4

Electroanatomical mapping for AV nodal reentrant tachycardia using CARTO™

Henry A. Chen, MD *& Henry H. Hsia,* MD

Clinical vignette

A 63-year-old woman with history of hypercholesterolemia was diagnosed with supraventricular tachycardia (SVT) and has had paroxysmal episodes of palpitations since her 30s. She has continued to have episodes despite beta-blocker therapy; she has had an increase in frequency of symptomatic episodes of palpitations and has had multiple emergency department visits and administration of adenosine for termination of the tachycardia.

Her cardiac evaluation includes a nuclear stress test and an echocardiogram that were normal with the exception of impaired diastolic relaxation.

A Holter monitor demonstrated evidence of supraventricular tachycardia at a heart rate of approximately 230–250 bpm (Figure 4.1).

Electrophysiology study and ablation

We were able to demonstrate dual AV node physiology, initiation of tachycardia by an atrial premature contraction with a jump to the slow pathway, concentric atrial activation with a V-A time of 30 ms, and a V-A-V response to right ventricular pacing were findings consistent with typical AV nodal reentrant tachycardia (Figure 4.2). The patient underwent successful RF ablation for slow pathway modification (Figure 4.3). Following ablation, the patient was no longer inducible for supraventricular tachycardia.

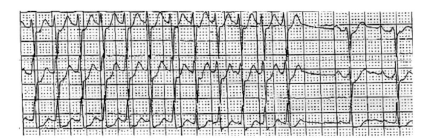

Figure 4.1   Holter monitor strip of tachycardia, demonstrating narrow complex tachycardia with rate approximately 250 bpm. Note that there are no visible P waves during tachycardia.

Electroanatomical Mapping, 1st edition. Edited by
A. Al-Ahmad, D. Callans, H. Hsia and A. Natale.
© 2008 Blackwell Publishing, ISBN: 9781405157025.

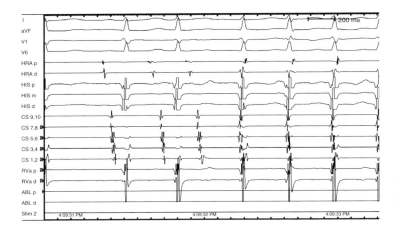

Figure 4.2 Spontaneous initiation of tachycardia with an atrial premature complex. Intracardiac electrograms demonstrated AV nodal reentrant tachycardia.

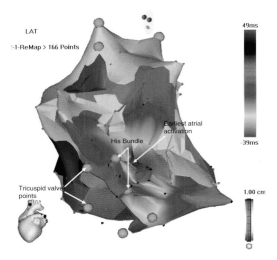

Figure 4.3 Activation map during tachycardia demonstrated atrial activation earliest (shown in the red area) in the fast pathway region. The remainder of the atrium is activated concentrically.

CHAPTER 5

Electroanatomical mapping for AV nodal reentrant tachycardia using NavX™

Henry A. Chen, MD *& Amin Al-Ahmad,* MD

Clinical vignette

A 45-year-old female with no known significant past medical history presented with episodes of palpitations that occurred approximately five to six times per week. Episodes last up to 30 min, and are associated with shortness of breath and palpitations. She was treated with beta-blockers, but has had incomplete reduction of episode frequency. She presented to the emergency department with severe palpitations and light-headedness and was found to have a heart rate of 150–160 bpm (Figure 5.1). The tachycardia terminated with adenosine. The echocardiogram demonstrated no significant abnormalities and normal systolic function. She was referred for further evaluation and treatment.

Electrophysiology study and ablation

Electrode catheters were placed in the high right atrium, His bundle region, coronary sinus, and right ventricular apex. The patient had normal baseline characteristics. Dual AV nodal physiology was demonstrated. An atrial premature depolarization followed by a jump to the slow pathway induced tachycardia with cycle length of 400 ms (Figure 5.1). The V-A time in tachycardia

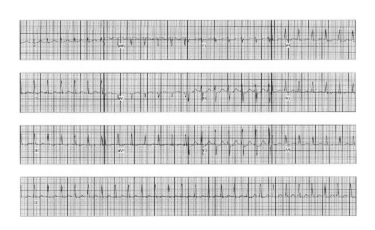

Figure 5.1 Tachycardia with cycle length of 400 ms.

Electroanatomical Mapping, 1st edition. Edited by
A. Al-Ahmad, D. Callans, H. Hsia and A. Natale.
© 2008 Blackwell Publishing, ISBN: 9781405157025.

was less than 70 ms. Other maneuvers, such as demonstration of a "V-A-V response" to right ventricular pacing (Figure 5.2) and para-hisian pacing (showing no evidence of accessory bypass tract) also supported the diagnosis of AV nodal reentrant tachycardia. An activation map was performed during tachycardia, which demonstrated early anterograde atrial activation in the slow pathway region as expected (Figures 5.3 and 5.4).

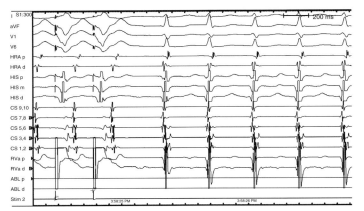

Figure 5.2 Entrainment pacing demonstrated V-A-V postpacing response, largely excluding atrial tachycardia. In addition, V-A time in tachycardia is less than 70 ms, consistent with AV nodal reentrant tachycardia.

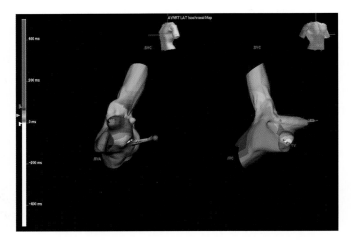

Figure 5.3 Activation pattern of tachycardia demonstrated concentric earliest atrial activation (white area) in the slow pathway region.

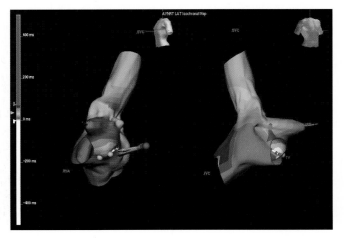

Figure 5.4 After electrophysiology study and activation mapping were performed, cryoablation lesions (yellow dots) were delivered to the slow pathway region. Following ablation, the tachycardia was no longer inducible.

6

CHAPTER 6

Slow pathway ablation

Robert Schweikert, MD, *Luigi Di Biase,*MD *& Andrea Natale,* MD

Clinical vignette

This case is a 51-year-old male with recurrent drug-refractory symptomatic narrow-complex tachycardia. This tachycardia was adenosine sensitive. The patient has no significant cardiac disease.

Electrophysiological study and ablation

Electrophysiological study demonstrated the tachycardia to be atrioventricular nodal reentrant tachycardia (AVNRT) (Figure 6.1). Using an anatomical and electrogram-guided approach, the atrioventricular (AV) nodal slow pathway region was mapped in sinus rhythm with a remote magnetic navigation system (Stereotaxis, St. Louis, MO). Locations at which a His potential was recorded were collected into an electroanatomical mapping system and displayed as points or "tags" on the virtual image (Figure 6.2). Successful catheter ablation was performed with the Biosense Webster RMT 4-mm catheter using the Stereotaxis remote magnetic navigation system. After several

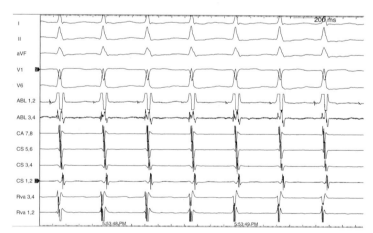

Figure 6.1 Electrograms from electrophysiological (EP) study in patient with recurrent, medically refractory supraventricular tachycardia. Leads I, II, aVF, V1 and V6, ablation/mapping catheter distal (ABL 1,2) and proximal (ABL 3,4) at His position, coronary sinus (CS) electrograms (CS 7,8 proximal to CS1,2 distal), right ventricular apex (RVa) catheter proximal (RVa 3,4), and distal (RVa 1,2). Note the simultaneous atrial and ventricular activation with very short V-A time consistent with AVNRT.

Electroanatomical Mapping, 1st edition. Edited by
A. Al-Ahmad, D. Callans, H. Hsia and A. Natale.
© 2008 Blackwell Publishing, ISBN: 9781405157025.

radiofrequency (RF) lesions were unsuccessful at sites more distant from the His region, more superior sites were explored. There was accelerated junctional rhythm during ablation at the successful site, which was found to be 7 mm from the most inferior portion of the "His cloud" on the electroanatomical map (Figure 6.2). After ablation, there was no longer inducible tachycardia. Figure 6.2 also demonstrates that the electrograms recorded

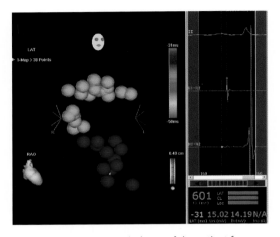

Figure 6.2 Electroanatomical map of the patient from Figure 6.1, showing an right anterior oblique (RAO) projection of location points marked from the position of the mapping catheter during sinus rhythm. The yellow points indicate those points at which a His bundle electrogram was recorded, thus creating the so-called His cloud, representing the extent of the region of the His bundle. The red points indicate those points at which RF ablation lesions were delivered. Note that the successful ablation site was at one of the highest ablation points, just 7 mm from the lowest extent of the His bundle region.

from the mapping/ablation catheter, in the slow pathway region, consists of a small amplitude atrial electrogram and a large amplitude ventricular electrogram. Catheter ablation of AV nodal slow pathway carries a low, but not insignificant, risk of heart block (0.5–2%), and different methods have been suggested in order to reduce these complications. The value of the creation of a detailed electroanatomical map of the His region is demonstrated in this case, as the successful ablation site required delivery of lesions closer to the His region than typically encountered. Note that the figure clearly demonstrates that the His bundle region is not a discrete point but rather a region that spans several centimeters from anterosuperior to posteroinferior. The advantages of the electroanatomical map in this case are several. The map provides a fairly detailed information regarding the location and extent of the His bundle region and its relative position to the potential ablation sites. The system allows real-time display of the mapping/ablation catheter on this map such that the catheter position may be tracked during the mapping and ablation procedure without the use of fluoroscopy. This is beneficial over the use of fluoroscopy alone for tracking the catheter position and monitoring its position relative to the His bundle region. Not evident in the illustrations was the additional benefit of the remote magnetic navigation system, which allowed manipulation of the mapping/ablation catheter from a remote console, including precise movements, to provide detailed mapping information for the His region and appropriate and stable positioning for the successful ablation site.

CHAPTER 7

Electroanatomical mapping for right-sided accessory pathway

Henry A. Chen, MD *& Amin Al-Ahmad,* MD

Clinical vignette

A 38-year-old man with Wolff–Parkinson–White syndrome and palpitations over the past 15 years presented with increasing episodes of palpitations. He has had multiple ER visits within the past 6 months for a narrow complex tachycardia at approximately 190 bpm, which was consistently terminated with adenosine. In the past the patient had been able to terminate episodes with Valsalva maneuvers. The patient elected to have electrophysiological study and ablation.

Electrophysiology study and ablation

Electrode catheters were placed in the high right atrium, His bundle region, coronary sinus, and right ventricular apex. Baseline intervals showed a short H-V time. Ventricular pacing revealed retrograde right-sided accessory pathway conduction (Figure 7.1). Supraventricular tachycardia was easily induced with an atrial premature depolarization (Figure 7.2). Electrophysiological observations (including advancement of atrial activity with a

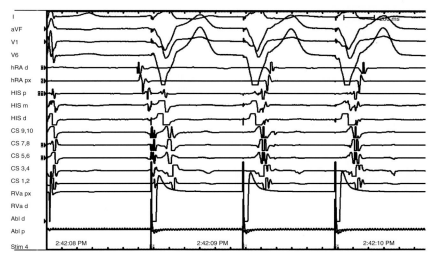

Figure 7.1   Right ventricular pacing demonstrated concentric retrograde atrial activation pattern.

Electroanatomical Mapping, 1st edition. Edited by
A. Al-Ahmad, D. Callans, H. Hsia and A. Natale.
© 2008 Blackwell Publishing, ISBN: 9781405157025.

ventricular premature depolarization [VPD] delivered during His bundle refractoriness and a "V-A-V" postventricular pacing response) supported the diagnosis of atrioventricular tachycardia. The retrograde atrial conduction pattern and the observation of no change in V-A time with left bundle branch block (LBBB) were consistent with location of the accessory pathway on the right (Figure 7.3).

By outlining the right atrial endocardial surface with a mapping catheter, an anatomical shell was created with the three-dimensional mapping system. Activation mapping was performed along the tricuspid isthmus, and the site of earliest activation during tachycardia was identified (Figures 7.4 and 7.5).

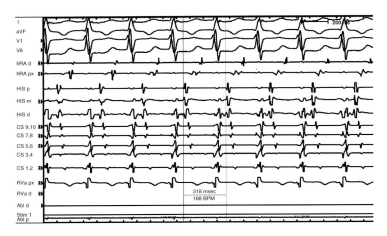

Figure 7.2 Supraventricular tachycardia.

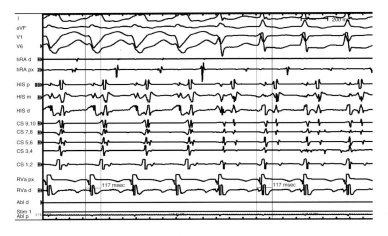

Figure 7.3 No change in V-A time with LBBB during tachycardia.

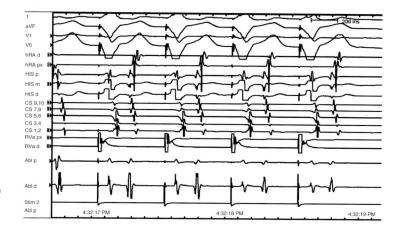

Figure 7.4 Activation mapping with the catheter positioned at the septal aspect of tricuspid annulus. Note the timing of the electrogram of the distal ablation catheter is slightly ahead of the earliest atrial electrogram.

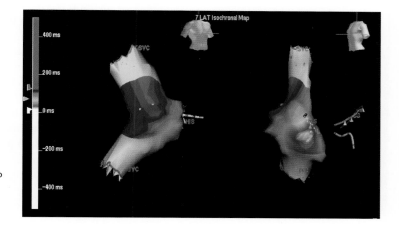

Figure 7.5 Electroanatomical mapping showed earliest retrograde atrial activation in the low right atrium along the septal aspect of the tricuspid annulus (white area). After a lesion was delivered at this site, there was no further evidence of bypass tract conduction and the tachycardia was not inducible.

CHAPTER 8

Ablation of an accessory pathway: endocardial and epicardial mapping

Robert Schweikert, MD *Luigi Di Biase*, MD *&*
Andrea Natale, MD, FACC, FHRS

Clinical vignette

A 40-year-old male was experiencing recurrent, medically refractory supraventricular tachycardia (SVT). A previous electrophysiology (EP) study had demonstrated the presence of a concealed left free wall accessory pathway and inducible orthodromic atrioventricular reciprocating tachycardia. Catheter ablation was unsuccessful and the pathway was considered to be potentially epicardial.

Electrophysiology study and ablation

A repeat EP study confirmed the presence of the left free wall accessory pathway, and activation mapping during tachycardia was performed endocardially and epicardially via a percutaneous pericardial approach. Endocardial sites were found to be earlier than epicardial sites (Figures 8.1 and 8.2), and catheter ablation on the atrial side of the mitral annulus from a trans-septal endocardial approach was successfully performed using an open irrigation catheter ablation system. Note that the electrograms from the mapping/ablation catheter (M1–M2, Figure 8.1) at the successful site demonstrating continuous electrical activity with fused ventricular and atrial electrograms. Although the accessory pathway was not ablated epicardially, this case illustrates the value of the additional dimension added by electroanatomical mapping from both an epicardial and endocardial approach. The epicardial map provides complimentary and additional information to the endocardial map, confirming the fact that the best site for ablation was indeed endocardial. In addition, the electroanatomical map provides a nonfluoroscopic means of tracking the real-time position of the mapping/ablation catheter displayed within the activation map. At any given point the position of the catheter may be recorded into the system represented by a "tag". Figure 8.3 shows an example of this, with the red dot representing the location of the catheter tip during delivery of a radiofrequency ablation lesion. The advantage of this location recording is that the catheter may be guided back to this point at any time after it is recorded, which is particularly valuable if the ablation catheter moves prematurely from the ablation site. In this manner, the catheter may be guided back to the location of the accessory pathway even after the pathway has been temporarily ablated so that more definitive and effective lesions may be delivered for successful ablation. Electroanatomical mapping has facilitated the localization of various arrhythmia substrates in addition to tracking the real-time positions of the mapping/ablation catheter.

Electroanatomical Mapping, 1st edition. Edited by
A. Al-Ahmad, D. Callans, H. Hsia and A. Natale.
© 2008 Blackwell Publishing, ISBN: 9781405157025.

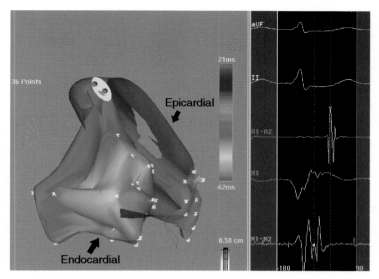

Figure 8.1 Endo-epicardial electroanatomical map (left anterior oblique [LAO] cranial view) and intracardiac electrograms from a patient with recurrent symptomatic SVT and a failed ablation attempt from an endocardial approach. EP study demonstrated a concealed accessory pathway. Endo-epicardial mapping was performed, and the figure shows the epicardial activation map superimposed over the endocardial activation map. The earliest activation was demonstrated endocardially at the left lateral mitral annulus and catheter ablation at this site was successful (note electrograms from mapping/ablation catheter M1–M2 at successful site).

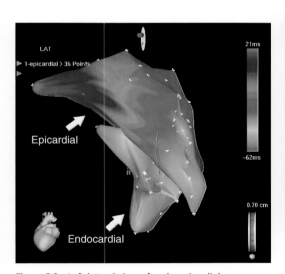

Figure 8.2 Left lateral view of endo-epicardial electroanatomical map.

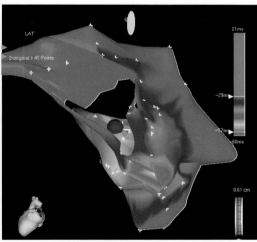

Figure 8.3 Endo-epicardial electroanatomical map (left posterior oblique view) demonstrating the site of successful catheter ablation on the endocardial map indicated by the red tag.

CHAPTER 9

Focal atrial tachycardia

Daejoon Anh, MD *& Henry H. Hsia,* MD

Clinical vignette

A 48-year-old female presented with a history of frequent paroxysmal palpitations since the age of 14. Surface electrocardiogram suggested long-RP supraventricular tachycardia at 135 bpm. A 12-lead rhythm strip performed during carotid sinus massage produced a transient atrioventricular block unveiling underlying atrial tachyarrhythmia (arrows, Figure 9.1).

Electrophysiologic study and ablation

Electrophysiology study with standard pacing maneuvers confirmed focal atrial tachycardia as the mechanism. Electroanatomic activation mapping of the right atrium during tachycardia with NAVX demonstrated the area immediately lateral to the coronary sinus ostium as the earliest point of activation (Figure 9.2), where the local electrogram was 40 ms prior to the onset of surface P wave (Figure 9.3). Application of radiofrequency energy at the earliest point of activation eliminated the tachycardia within 1.8 s. Note the decrease in local electrogram amplitude in the distal ablation channel (ABL d) just prior to the termination of the atrial tachycardia.

Electroanatomical Mapping, 1st edition. Edited by
A. Al-Ahmad, D. Callans, H. Hsia and A. Natale.
© 2008 Blackwell Publishing, ISBN: 9781405157025.

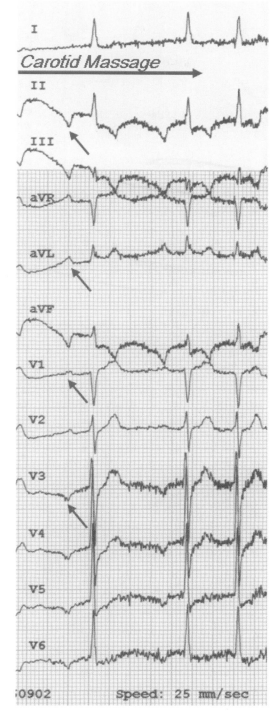

Figure 9.1 The 12-lead rhythm strip of atrial tachycardia recorded during carotid massage shows uninterrupted atrial activity clearly defining P waves. The P-wave morphology was similar to that of counterclockwise cavotricuspid isthmus atrial flutter, whose exit from the isthmus is similar to the focal origin of this atrial tachycardia.

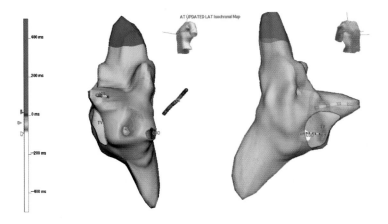

Figure 9.2   NAVX activation map of the atrial tachycardia in left anterior oblique (LAO) and right anterior oblique (RAO) views. The earliest point of activation is represented by the white-colored isochrone. The ablation catheter position shown in the figure was the successful ablation position. His and coronary sinus catheters and coronary sinus ostium (CSO) are also shown.

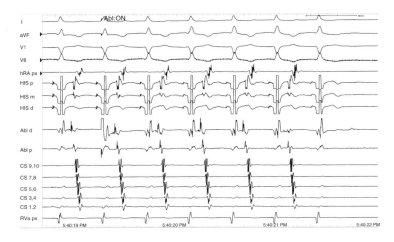

Figure 9.3   Bipolar electrogram from the successful ablation site is shown. The local electrogram demonstrated activation 40 ms prior to the onset of surface P wave. Application of radiofrequency energy at this site resulted in the elimination of atrial tachycardia within 1.8 s.

CHAPTER 10

Electroanatomical mapping for right para-hisian atrial tachycardia

Rupa Bala, MD

Clinical vignette

A 51-year-old male with a history of ulcerative colitis and palpitations for many years treated with beta-blockers was referred to our institution for electrophysiology study and ablation due to increasingly severe and frequent episodes. Echo-cardiogram revealed a structurally normal heart with preserved ejection fraction. The ECG revealed a short-RP tachycardia with a tachycardia cycle length of 320 ms.

Electrophysiologic study and ablation

An electrophysiology study was performed and induced a supraventricular tachyarrhythmia (SVT) that was consistent with an atrial tachycardia by pacing maneuvers and was adenosine sensitive (Figures 10.1 and 10.2). The right para-hisian, left para-hisian, and noncoronary cusp were mapped extensively and the site of earliest activation was found to be in the right para-hisian

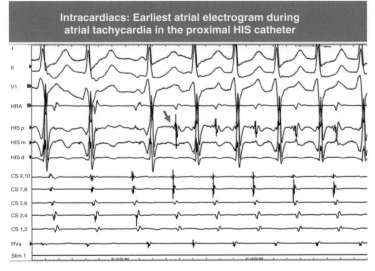

Intracardiacs: Earliest atrial electrogram during atrial tachycardia in the proximal HIS catheter

Figure 10.1 Intracardiac recordings of the atrial tachycardia are shown. ECG leads I, II, V1, high right atrial (HRA) catheter, His catheter (HIS) with proximal, middle, and distal poles, coronary sinus (CS) catheter with proximal to distal poles, and right ventricular apex (RVA) catheter are shown. The earliest atrial electrogram during tachycardia is seen in the proximal His catheter.

Electroanatomical Mapping, 1st edition. Edited by
A. Al-Ahmad, D. Callans, H. Hsia and A. Natale.
© 2008 Blackwell Publishing, ISBN: 9781405157025.

region (Figure 10.3). At the site of earliest activation, cryoablation was used to successfully terminate the focal, adenosine-sensitive atrial tachycardia. The PR interval remained unchanged. Subsequent, programmed stimulation on and off

of isoproterenol failed to reinitiate the tachycardia. Six months after the procedure, the patient continues to do well without recurrence of atrial tachycardia off of medications.

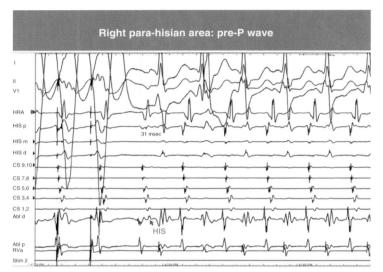

Figure 10.2   Ventricular pacing is used to separate the P wave from the preceding T wave in order to measure the activation time from the distal pole of the ablation catheter (Abl d) to the onset of the P wave. Mapping in the right para-hisian area with a 4-mm CARTO™ catheter showed that the earliest activation time was 31-ms "pre-P wave". At this site, cryoablation was used to terminate the tachycardia. Note the HIS deflection on the ablation catheter.

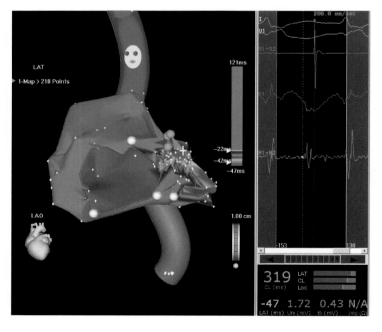

Figure 10.3   Right atrial activation map during adenosine-sensitive atrial tachycardia. Note that the site of earliest activation is located in the right para-hisian region. The yellow tags denote "HIS" deflections and the white "x" marks the area that corresponds to the electrogram on the distal pole of the mapping catheter (M1–M2) in the right window. Note the "HIS" deflection on the mapping catheter at the site of earliest activation.

CHAPTER 11

Right atrial tachycardia after ablation for inappropriate sinus tachycardia

David Callans, MD, FACC, FHRS

Clinical vignette

A 26-year-old woman had a history of severe palpitations with presyncope and chest pain; ambulatory monitoring led to a presumptive diagnosis of inappropriate sinus tachycardia. After failure of medical management, she underwent sinus node modification. After ablation, there was an abrupt reduction in resting heart rate, as well as maximal heart rate on isoproterenol challenge. The P-wave morphology in sinus rhythm changed, and was negative in lead III.

She was well for 18 months, but then complained of palpitations once again, but without presyncope or chest pain. Monitoring showed a paroxysmal narrow complex tachycardia. She returned for electrophysiologic study.

Electrophysiologic study and ablation

EnSite Array mapping during resting rhythm showed a mid-low crista location of the earliest activation (again, note the negative P wave in lead III) (Figure 11.1). The maximal heart rate on 10 μg of isoproterenol was only 145 bpm, and did not reproduce her symptoms. Programmed atrial stimulation induced an atrial tachycardia, which was mapped to near the ostium of the coronary sinus and successfully ablated (Figure 11.2).

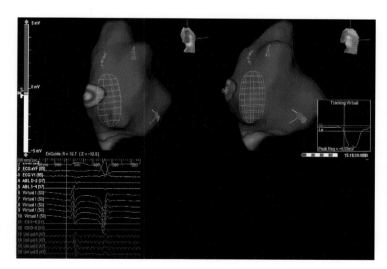

Figure 11.1 EnSite Array mapping of resting rhythm that originates from the crista terminalis.

Electroanatomical Mapping, 1st edition. Edited by
A. Al-Ahmad, D. Callans, H. Hsia and A. Natale.
© 2008 Blackwell Publishing, ISBN: 9781405157025.

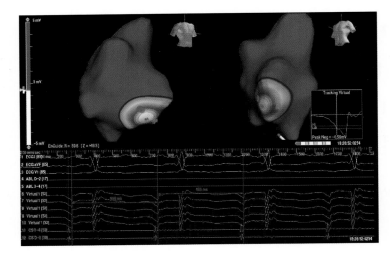

Figure 11.2 Induced atrial tachycardia with a site of origin near the ostium of the coronary sinus.

CHAPTER 12

Inappropriate sinus tachycardia

Greg Feld, MD

Clinical vignette

The patient is a 55-year-old female, with a history of AV nodal reentrant tachycardia (AVNRT), who underwent three separate slow pathway ablation attempts, including ablation within the coronary sinus ostium to finally cure the AVNRT. Subsequently, the patient had no arrhythmias until she developed inappropriate sinus tachycardia (IAST). Over the past 3 years she has had resting heart rates as high as 120 bpm and exercise heart rates as high as 200 bpm (Figure 12.1). The patient failed to respond to treatment with numerous beta-blockers, in part due to side effects. The patient also has a history of hypertension, nephrolithiasis, and hereditary spherocytosis treated by splenectomy.

Electrophysiology study and ablation

The patient therefore underwent electrophysiology (EP) study and attempted modification of the sinus node for the treatment of IAST. The diagnostic study revealed no evidence of dual AV nodal physiology or inducible AVNRT. At baseline a sinus tachycardia was noted. Mapping with the EnSite balloon array revealed earliest atrial activation at the junction of the superior vena cava and anterior right atrium near the base of the atrial appendage (Figure 12.2). Ablation in this region eliminated IAST, and the patient developed a subsidiary atrial rhythm at a rate of 60 bpm (Figure 12.3), the origin of which was mapped to the crista terminalis, approximately two-thirds of the way down from

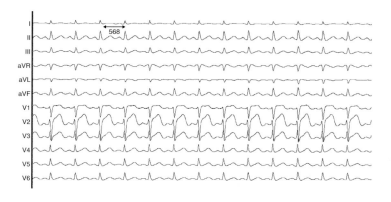

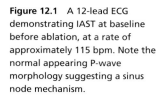

Figure 12.1 A 12-lead ECG demonstrating IAST at baseline before ablation, at a rate of approximately 115 bpm. Note the normal appearing P-wave morphology suggesting a sinus node mechanism.

Electroanatomical Mapping, 1st edition. Edited by
A. Al-Ahmad, D. Callans, H. Hsia and A. Natale.
© 2008 Blackwell Publishing, ISBN: 9781405157025.

the superior to the inferior vena cava (Figure 12.4). Ablation was performed with an EP Technologies Blazer™ 8-mm-tip catheter, at a power of 60 W and temperature of 55°C for up to 60 s during each energy application. Pacing at 10 mA and 5 ms was performed before ablation to ensure lack of phrenic nerve stimulation. A total of 18 radiofrequency energy applications were required to eliminate

IAST. During isoproterenol infusion at 5 mcg/min following ablation, the highest sinus rate was 90 bpm, and there was a shift in earliest site of activation to the base of the right atrial appendage, distal to the site of ablation (Figure 12.5). During 1-month follow-up since ablation, the patient has had no further IAST and has maintained a normal heart rate at rest and during exercise.

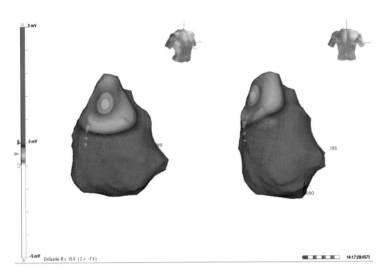

Figure 12.2 Ensite™ balloon array voltage/activation map of the right atrium at baseline, demonstrating the site of earliest activation during IAST (white area), near the junction of the superior vena cava and right atrial appendage, the expected location of the sinus node. CSO = coronary sinus ostium; HIS = His bundle.

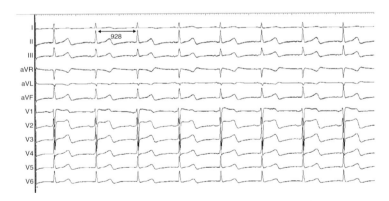

Figure 12.3 A 12-lead ECG following radiofrequency ablation of earliest site of activation during IAST, demonstrating a slow sinus rate to near 60 bpm at rest. A P-wave morphology suggests a lower atrial origin of the pacemaker activity.

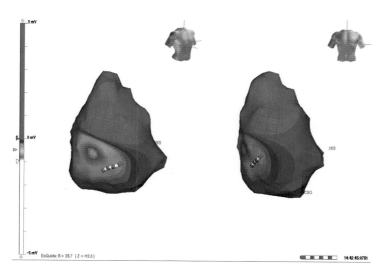

Figure 12.4 Ensite™ balloon array voltage/activation map of the right atrium following ablation of IAST, demonstrating the site of origin (white area) of the subsidiary pacemaker activity approximately two-thirds of the way down the crista terminalis from the superior vena cava. The average heart rate was 60 bpm following ablation. CSO = coronary sinus ostium; HIS = His bundle.

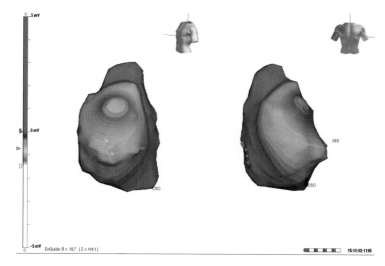

Figure 12.5 Ensite™ balloon array voltage/activation map of the right atrium following ablation of IAST, during isoproterenol infusion at 5 mcg/min, demonstrating the site of origin (white area) of the subsidiary pacemaker activity at the base of the right atrial appendage, distal to the ablation site near the sinus node. The heart rate reached a maximum of 90 bpm during isoproterenol infusion. CSO = coronary sinus ostium; HIS = His bundle.

CHAPTER 13

Focal left atrial tachycardia

Sumeet K. Mainigi, MD

Clinical vignette

The patient is a 37-year-old female physician with palpitations beginning a year prior to her procedure. Treatment with beta-blockers was unsuccessful in relieving her symptoms. After several months, she underwent an electrophysiologic study at another institution, which demonstrated a likely para-hisian atrial tachycardia, although it was difficult to induce and only short episodes were observed during the procedure (Figure 13.1). The procedure was aborted because of concern over the risk of conduction block. The patient subsequently failed flecainide and propafenone and was referred for repeat ablation

(a) (b)

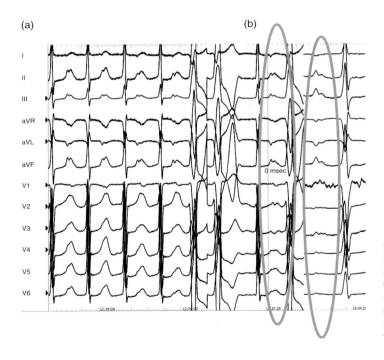

Figure 13.1 (a) An atrial tachycardia (variable cycle length between 380 and 410 ms) was easily induced with atrial burst pacing. The P-wave morphology is identified and suggests a left atrial site. (b) The P-wave morphology is shown at a faster paper speed.

Electroanatomical Mapping, 1st edition. Edited by
A. Al-Ahmad, D. Callans, H. Hsia and A. Natale.
© 2008 Blackwell Publishing, ISBN: 9781405157025.

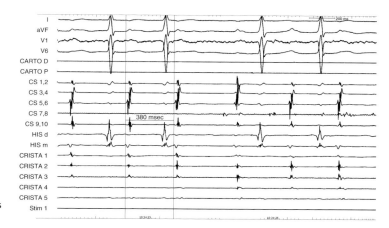

Figure 13.2 The atrial activation pattern demonstrates early activation along the coronary sinus catheter.

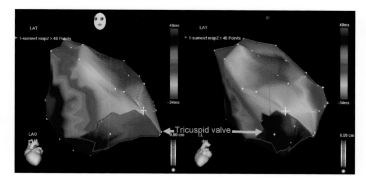

Figure 13.3 Left anterior oblique (left) and left lateral (right) electroanatomic activation maps are shown of the right atrium. Diffuse septal activation is observed.

using cryotherapy. Physical examination and transthoracic echocardiogram were unremarkable.

Electrophysiology study and ablation

An electroanatomic activation map of the right atrium was created and demonstrated diffuse activation along the interatrial septum, earliest activation was along the coronary sinus catheter (Figures 13.2 and 13.3). Given this diffuse activation, a left atrial tachycardia source was suspected. A trans-septal puncture was performed and the mapping catheter was advanced into the left atrium. An activation map was created of the left atrium (Figure 13.4). Placement of the right atrial and left atrial maps together demonstrates the right atrium, which is passively activated from the left atrium. The earliest activation was from the base of the left atrial appendage near the mitral annulus. Radiofrequency ablation at this site terminated the arrhythmia (Figure 13.5).

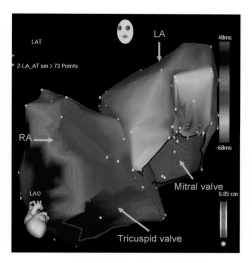

Figure 13.4 An activation map is created of the left atrium (LA) and placed in the appropriate position next to the right atrium (RA). The RA demonstrates relatively late activation in comparison to the earlier LA. The earliest site of activation appears to be at the base of the left atrial appendage, near the mitral valve.

(a)

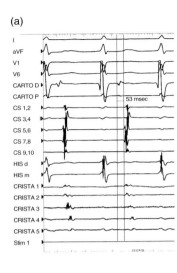

(b)

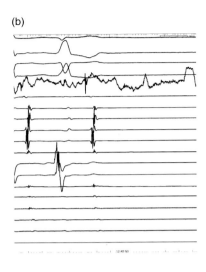

Figure 13.5   (a) The site of earliest atrial activation. (b) A radiofrequency lesion delivered at this site resulted in termination of the tachycardia.

CHAPTER 14

Electroanatomical mapping of right atrial tricuspid annulus atrial tachycardia

Pirooz Mofrad, MD *& Henry Hsia,* MD

Clinical vignette

A 61-year-old male with past medical history of hypercholesterolemia was referred to the electrophysiology service for palpitations. He has a history of paroxysmal, symptomatic supraventricular tachycardia at 160 bpm (Figure 14.1). He had no structural heart disease and a stress nuclear perfusion test was normal. Given a history of frequent symptomatic episodes, the patient underwent electrophysiology testing with electroanatomic mapping using the CARTO™ system.

Electrophysiology study and ablation

With atrial burst pacing, the patient had easily inducible atrial tachycardia with a tachycardia cycle length of 400 ms (Figure 14.2). Electroanatomical activation mapping was performed using the CARTO™ system. Earliest fragmented atrial activation was noted at a focal site along the lateral tricuspid annulus during sustained atrial tachycardia (Figure 14.3). Using the CARTO™ electroanatomical mapping system, an activation map of the right atrium was constructed during atrial tachycardia (Figure 14.4).

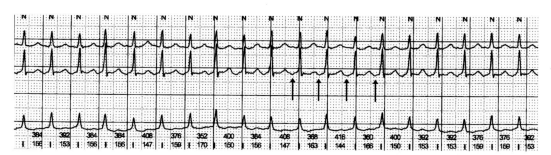

Figure 14.1 Outpatient Holter demonstrated episodes of supraventricular tachyarrhythmia (SVT) at approximately 160 bpm, with preceding atrial activity suggestive of an ectopic atrial tachycardia (labeled by arrows).

Electroanatomical Mapping, 1st edition. Edited by
A. Al-Ahmad, D. Callans, H. Hsia and A. Natale.
© 2008 Blackwell Publishing, ISBN: 9781405157025.

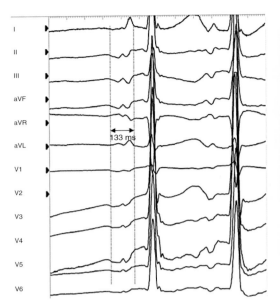

Figure 14.2 Comparison of the P-wave morphology and duration between the normal sinus rhythm (~122 ms), and that during atrial tachycardia (~133 ms). The broad, notched P waves with a predominately negative precordial transition suggested the site of origin originated from the anterior lateral right atrium.

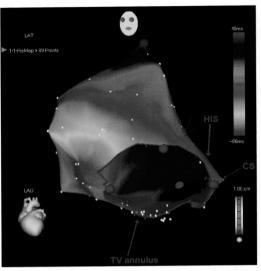

Figure 14.4 LAO view of activation mapping performed during sustained atrial tachycardia with earliest activation seen at the 8 o'clock position in LAO. Focal activation with concentric wave front propagation suggested a focal automatic atrial tachycardia. Radiofrequency ablation lesions were directed to this site with successful termination and noninducibility of the focal atrial tachycardia. TV refers to tricuspid valve and CS refers to coronary sinus os.

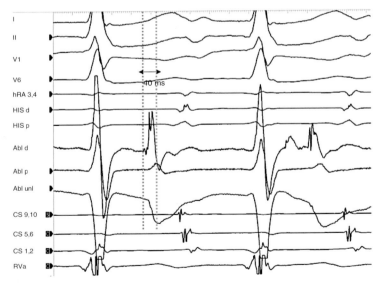

Figure 14.3 Activation mapping at 8 o'clock in left anterior oblique (LAO) position on the tricuspid annulus with local atrial activation "spike" was present that precedes the surface P-wave onset by 40 ms. Negative unipolar atrial recordings were also observed.

CHAPTER 15

Electroanatomical mapping of a left-sided atrial tachycardia

Kevin Makati, MD *& N. A. Mark Estes III,* MD

Clinical vignette

The patient is a 34-year-old female with a long history of symptomatic atrial tachycardia failing verapamil and quinidine (Figure 15.1). An attempt at radiofrequency ablation was made 6 years prior to her presentation without success. She was brought back to the electrophysiology lab for another attempt at ablation.

Electrophysiology study and ablation

The patient was brought to the electrophysiology laboratory for electroanatomic mapping of the atrial tachycardia focus. The right atrium was mapped quickly using the CARTO™ system (Figure 15.2). The site of earliest atrial activation appears to be the more distal coronary sinus suggesting a

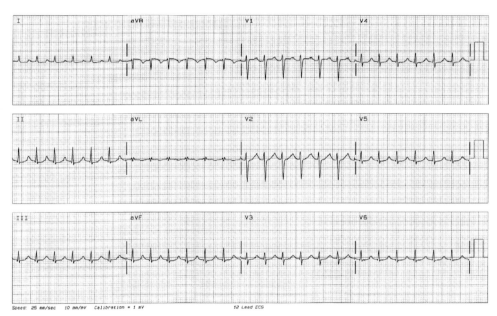

Figure 15.1 A 12-lead electrocardiogram of the atrial tachycardia. The P-wave axis is helpful to localize the optimal site for ablation; however, judging the axis is difficult if the P wave is buried within the T wave as in this example.

Electroanatomical Mapping, 1st edition. Edited by
A. Al-Ahmad, D. Callans, H. Hsia and A. Natale.
© 2008 Blackwell Publishing, ISBN: 9781405157025.

left-sided tachycardia (Figure 15.3). The left atrium is mapped after trans-septal puncture. The site of earliest activation appeared to be close to the left inferior pulmonary vein (Figure 15.4). After one lesion in this area, the tachycardia terminated.

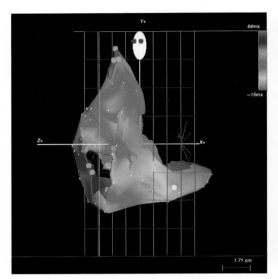

Figure 15.2 Electroanatomic map of the right atrium in left anterior oblique (LAO) projection. The site of earliest activation appears to be within the coronary sinus, but these points precede the reference catheter electrogram by only 15 ms, suggesting that the tachycardia focus has not been mapped.

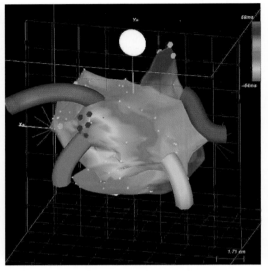

Figure 15.4 Electroanatomic map of the left atrium shown posteriorly. The site of earliest activation is −64 ms and is located adjacent to the inferior left pulmonary vein. Ablation in this area resulted in termination of the tachycardia.

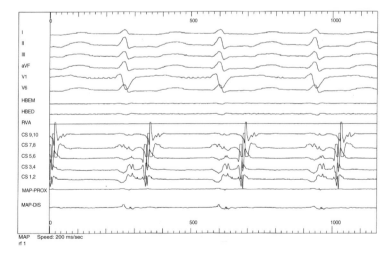

Figure 15.3 Intracardiac recording during atrial tachycardia. The earliest activation on the decapolar catheter within the coronary sinus is bipole 1,2, suggesting a left atrial focus.

CHAPTER 16

Focal atrial tachycardia

John Triedman, MD

Clinical vignette

The patient is a 17-year-old athletic young woman with a long-standing history of palpitations and documented narrow-complex tachycardia Episodes have persisted despite prophylactic medical therapy with verapamil. She had a structurally and functionally normal heart by echocardiogram. Resting electrocardiogram demonstrated non-pre-excited sinus rhythm. The pre-ablation working diagnosis was AV nodal reentrant tachycardia (AVNRT) based on her age and clinical presentation.

Electrophysiology study and ablation

The patient was initially in sinus rhythm. During placement of electrophysiology (EP) catheters, atrial tachycardia at cycle length 410 ms with variable conduction occurred (Figure 16.1). This tachycardia terminated spontaneously, but was easily reproducibly initiated and terminated with single atrial extrastimulus. Mapping was initially performed via measurement of postpacing interval at multiple sites. Mapping of the right and left (via patent foramen ovale) suggested a lateral right

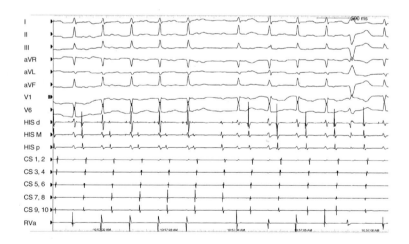

Figure 16.1 Slow atrial tachycardia induced and terminated easily by atrial extrastimuli.

Electroanatomical Mapping, 1st edition. Edited by
A. Al-Ahmad, D. Callans, H. Hsia and A. Natale.
© 2008 Blackwell Publishing, ISBN: 9781405157025.

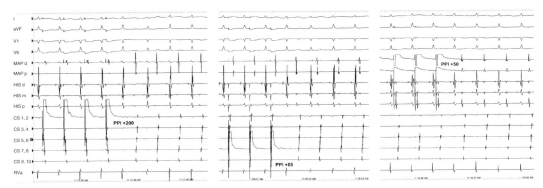

Figure 16.2   Postpacing intervals (PPIs) taken at three sites in the right atrium. Left panel: Pacing from distal CS (CS 1,2), first PPI was +200 ms. Middle panel: Pacing from proximal CS (CS 9,10), first PPI was +85 ms. Right panel: Pacing from high lateral right atrium (Map d), first PPI was +50 ms.

atrial origin of the tachycardia (Figure 16.2). Electroanatomical (CARTO™) mapping was performed next. The CARTO™ mapping revealed a single discrete focus of origin, at the anterolateral tricuspid annulus (Figure 16.3). The focal origin of the tachycardia, in combination with the easily initiation of the tachycardia with atrial extrastimuli, indicated that this was a focal atrial reentrant tachycardia. Ablation was performed at the anterolateral tricuspid annulus (Figure 16.4). Acute success (termination of tachycardia) occurred ~3 s into the first radiofrequency (RF) lesion (Figure 16.5). Attempts to reproduce the location at the AV annulus revealed that there was a significant discrepancy in the location of the AV annulus, presumably due to changes in atrial loading in sinus rhythm. An additional four RF lesions were made on the AV groove in the same area (Figure 16.6), with the CARTO™ catheter stabilized by an SR-2 long sheath. Following these ablations, the atrial tachycardia could not be induced. However, with progressive atrial stimulation, AH prolongation to 330 ms was noted, and a maximum of three beats of AVNRT could be induced on isoproterenol. A slow pathway modification was performed prior to finishing the case (Figure 16.7). It was initially assumed in this case that the atrial tachycardia, although of long cycle length for atrial flutter, was a spurious, nonclinical rhythm induced by catheter manipulation. However, its persistence and easy re-inducibility quickly suggested that it was in fact a clinically relevant ablation target.

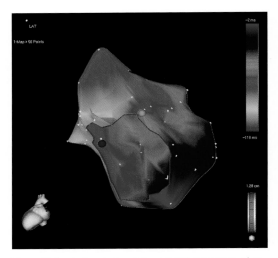

Figure 16.3   Left anterior oblique (LAO) projection of an electroanatomical activation map of the right atrium. The estimated tricuspid valve annulus as shown, with early activation in and the site of successful RF application the anterolateral aspect of the annulus. Orange tag marks the site of recorded His potential.

The postpacing interval was initially performed in the cavotricuspid isthmus, and once that was ruled out as a target, electroanatomical mapping was initiated to help refine the mapping of an atypical atrial focus. Focal reentrant tachycardias arising from the tricuspid annulus such as this one have been described, but their underlying mechanism and anatomic substrate is unknown.

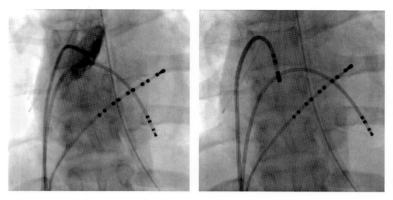

Figure 16.4 Anteroposterior (AP) fluoroscopy of the right atrial appendage and its relation to the successful ablation site.

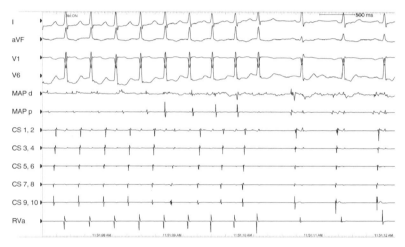

Figure 16.5 Termination of atrial tachycardia with ablation.

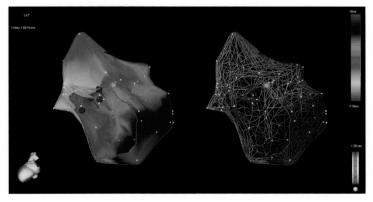

Figure 16.6 Additional applications of RF made in sinus rhythm are significantly deviated posteriorly for the former plane of the tricuspid annulus.

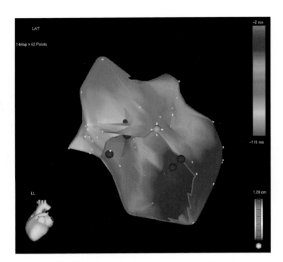

Figure 16.7 Additional lesions in posterior AV septum delineating site of slow pathway modification.

An interesting and important observation in this case is the discrepancy in catheter position recorded at the initial, successful ablation site, and the location of the AV groove, confirmed by analysis of local atrial and ventricular electrogram balance and corresponding to that site at which additional RF applications were made in sinus rhythm. Presumably, the marked discrepancy noted on the electroanatomical map (and also noted on fluoroscopy) represents the dynamic change in cardiac geometry associated with rhythm transition. Although this is a more dramatic shift than is commonly seen, in our lab experience, it is important to note that maps made of the same chamber in different rhythms may differ significantly.

CHAPTER 17

Ectopic atrial tachycardia

George Van Hare, MD

Clinical vignette

A 16-year-old male with a 2-year history of incessant ectopic atrial tachycardia despite treatment with two antiarrhythmic medications is referred for ablation. He has no other significant past medical history and his heart is structurally normal by echocardiogram. His 12-lead ECG P waves were upright in the inferior leads (Figure 17.1).

Electrophysiology study and ablation

The procedure was performed under local anesthesia and IV conscious sedation to avoid suppressing the ectopic focus. An isochronal activation map was acquired using NavX (Figure 17.2). The earliest activation was found at the summit of the interatrial septum (Figures 17.2 and 17.3). Delivery of radiofrequency energy in this location resulted in termination of the tachycardia.

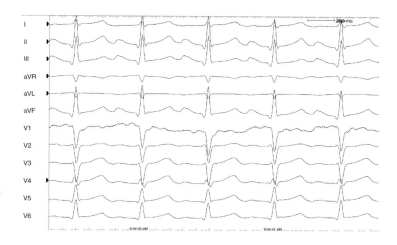

Figure 17.1 A 12-lead ECG of incessant atrial tachycardia. Note that the P waves are sinus-like but are somewhat flat in lead 1, and the PR interval is somewhat prolonged.

Electroanatomical Mapping, 1st edition. Edited by
A. Al-Ahmad, D. Callans, H. Hsia and A. Natale.
© 2008 Blackwell Publishing, ISBN: 9781405157025.

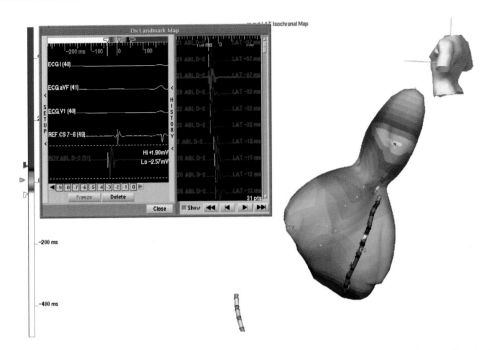

Figure 17.2 Isochronal activation map of the right atrium shows a simple activation pattern with the earliest local atrial activation found at the summit of the interatrial septum, where the local atrial activation preceded surface P wave by 35 ms.

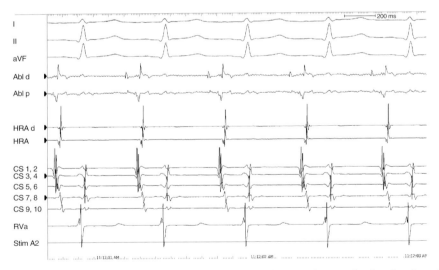

Figure 17.3 Intracardiac electrograms during atrial tachycardia, with ablation catheter at the site of earliest atrial activation, at the summit of the interatrial septum. The coronary sinus catheter was advanced deeply into the coronary sinus so that the distal electrode pair was at approximately 1:00 in left anterior oblique (LAO) view. Note the double potential recorded by the ablation catheter, with the earliest local atrial activation far in advance of the distal coronary sinus.

CHAPTER 18

Electroanatomical mapping for scar-based reentrant atrial tachycardia

Pirooz Mofrad, MD *& Amin Al-Ahmad,* MD

Clinical vignette

A 36-year-old female with a history of an atrial tachycardia was referred for recurrent episodes of tachycardia refractory to sotalol. She had an aortic valve replacement with mitral valve commissurotomy secondary to rheumatic heart disease. In addition, she suffered a primary ventricular fibrillation arrest in 2002 with subsequent implantable cardioverter defibrillator (ICD) placement. In 2004, an electrophysiology study was performed with a cavotricuspid isthmus ablation performed for typical right atrial flutter. She has had episodes of inappropriate ICD shocks secondary to her atrial tachyarrhythmia and has been experiencing increasing symptomatic palpitations (Figure 18.1).

Electrophysiology study and ablation

Baseline electrophysiology study was performed with a His, coronary sinus (CS 1,2 distally with

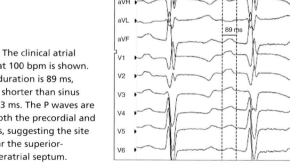

Figure 18.1 The clinical atrial tachycardia at 100 bpm is shown. The P-wave duration is 89 ms, considerably shorter than sinus P wave of 123 ms. The P waves are positive in both the precordial and inferior leads, suggesting the site of origin near the superior-posterior interatrial septum.

Electroanatomical Mapping, 1st edition. Edited by A. Al-Ahmad, D. Callans, H. Hsia and A. Natale. © 2008 Blackwell Publishing, ISBN: 9781405157025.

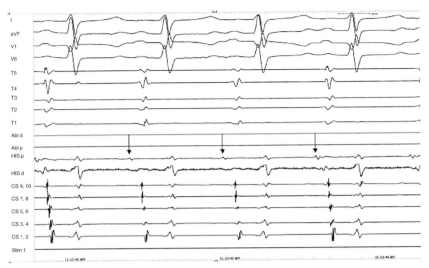

Figure 18.2   Atrial activation pattern during atrial tachycardia is shown with the earliest atrial activation located posterior to the His catheter position (with proximal earlier than distal) – denoted by arrows.

CS 9,10 at coronary sinus os), and an additional decapolar catheter (T1–T5) placed in the postero-lateral right atrium for activation mapping. The patient was easily inducible with atrial burst pacing and with isoproterenol infusion. The atrial tachy-cardia cycle length was approximately 600 ms.

Activation mapping during the atrial tachycardia was performed from the right atrium. The earliest atrial activation was mapped to the atrial septum, with a local electrogram to surface P wave time of 50 ms (Figure 18.2). An area of low voltage and scar encompassed portions of the mid- and superior interatrial septum (Figure 18.3). The atrial tachy-cardia was successfully entrained from sites in the mid- and superior posterior interatrial septum, at these sites of low-voltage and fragmented signals (Figure 18.4).

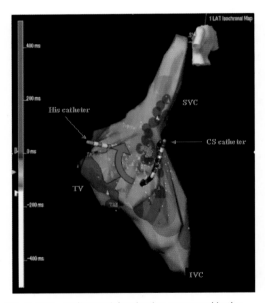

Figure 18.3   Earliest atrial activation was noted in the mid- to superior-posterior interatrial septum. Activation and entrainment mapping was consistent with a micro-reentrant circuit involving the atrial septum. Using entrain-ment techniques, a proposed isthmus site and exit site was identified, with excellent pace-maps in comparison to the atrial tachycardia P wave. The proposed circuit appeared to be along the inferior to superior atrial septum, along the area of the scar, with activation pattern as noted by the arrow. CS refers to coronary sinus, SVC refers to superior vena cava, IVC refers to inferior vena cava, and TV refers to tricuspid valve annulus.

(a)   (b)

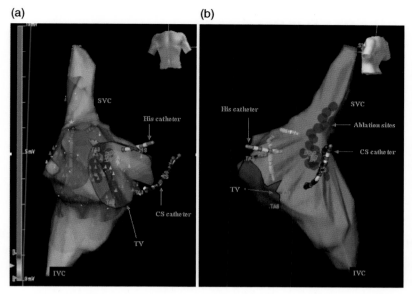

Figure 18.4   (a and b) The voltage map of the right atrium and interatrial septum with an area of low-voltage scar and fragmented signals. Multicomponent electrograms were recorded at the "isthmus" site. Linear ablation was performed from the junction of the RA-SVC (denoted by ablation dots in Panel B), transecting the scar including the exit and isthmus sites and successfully terminating the atrial tachycardia. CS refers to coronary sinus, SVC refers to superior vena cava, IVC refers to inferior vena cava, and TV refers to tricuspid valve annulus.

19 CHAPTER 19

Atrial flutter in a patient post Fontan

Riccardo Cappato, MD

Clinical vignette

DL is a 20-year-old boy with a double-inlet left ventricle who underwent Fontan-type surgery when he was 3 years old. When he was 15 years old, owing to recurrent episodes of atrial tachy-arrhythmia, he underwent Fontan conversion with the creation of a fenestrated intraatrial tunnel and atrial plasty. The postsurgical course was characterized by moderate desaturation that improved progressively.

Four weeks after discharge he developed incessant atrial tachycardia (Figure 19.1) associated with desaturation and moderate hypotension. At that time, intravenous and subsequently oral amiodarone failed to restore sinus rhythm. The patient was immediately referred to our center for catheter ablation of the arrhythmia substrate.

Electrophysiology study and ablation

An electrophysiological study was performed with two catheters advanced from the right femoral vein to the inferior vena cava and finally passed through the fenestration into the original right atrium. One diagnostic catheter, serving as reference and for backup pacing, was placed within the right atrium along the posterior-lateral wall, whereas a Navistar

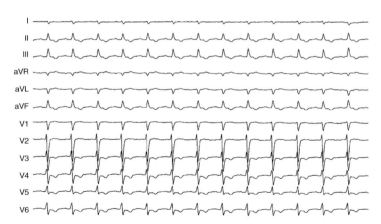

Figure 19.1 Incessant atrial tachycardia at 166 bpm, with 2:1 AV conduction.

Electroanatomical Mapping, 1st edition. Edited by
A. Al-Ahmad, D. Callans, H. Hsia and A. Natale.
© 2008 Blackwell Publishing, ISBN: 9781405157025.

catheter (CARTO™) was navigated inside the right atrium in search of critical areas for arrhythmia perpetuation (Figure 19.2). At the beginning of the procedure, the incessant atrial tachycardia presented with a cycle length of 360 ms. Electro-anatomical mapping was performed using a three-dimensional CARTO™ map. A macroreentrant circuit was identified in the right atrium with various areas of scar tissue (Figures 19.3 and 19.4). Multiple (up to 60) pulses of radiofrequency (RF) energy delivered at the posterior-lateral wall surrounding a protected isthmus of viable tissue with slow conduction ultimately succeeded in terminating atrial tachycardia (Figure 19.5). Finally, atrial tachycardia was no longer inducible after ablation either in basal conditions or under infusion of isoproterenol 2 mcg/kg/min (Figure 19.6).

During a follow-up of 5 years, the patient experienced two recurrences, both during an attempt to reduce therapy. Rhythm control is currently obtained under therapy with amiodarone (100 mg daily) and propanolol 2 mg/kg daily.

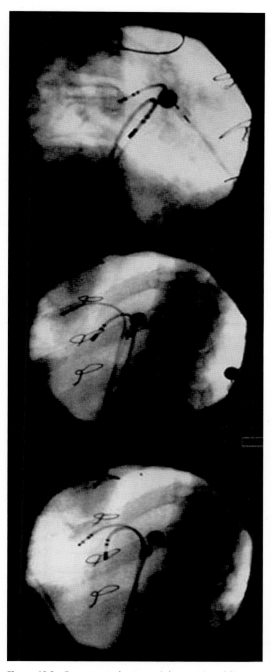

Figure 19.2 From top to bottom, right anterior oblique (RAO), anterior-posterior (AP), and left anterior oblique (LAO) projections showing the diagnostic and the map/ablation catheters advanced through the conduit fenestration in the right atrium. Note that the map/ablation catheter is positioned at the site of atrial tachycardia termination.

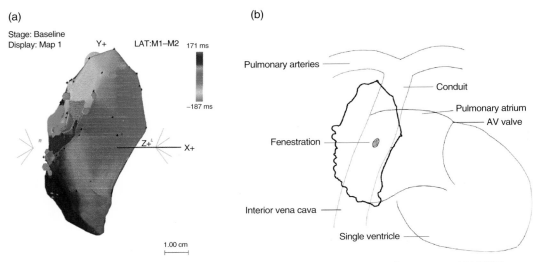

Figure 19.3   (a) Right inferior–anterior oblique projection showing the three-dimensional reconstructed CARTO™ map during atrial tachycardia. (b) The reconstructed right atrium is depicted (bold contours) in relationship with contiguous structures (light contours), including the artificial conduit connecting the inferior vena cava with the pulmonary arteries, the remaining atrium, the AV valve, and the single ventricle. Also depicted is the fenestration within the artificial conduit enabling the blood flow from within the conduit to enter the right atrium. Red dots identify sites of RF pulse delivery.

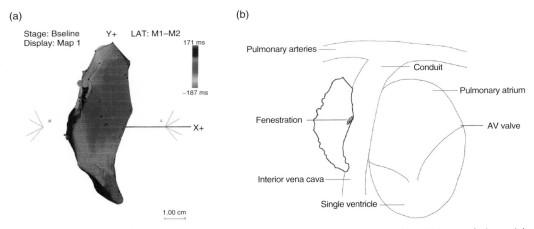

Figure 19.4   (a) Anterior–posterior projection showing the three-dimensional reconstructed CARTO™ map during atrial tachycardia. (b) The reconstructed right atrium is depicted (bold contours) in relationship with contiguous structures (light contours) as outlined in Figure 19.2.

(a)

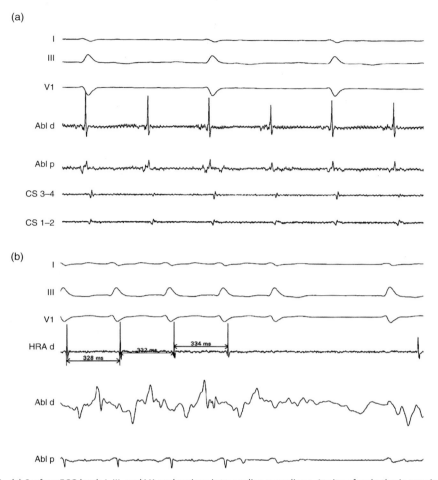

Figure 19.5 (a) Surface ECG leads I, III, and V1 and various intracardiac recordings. At site of arrhythmia termination, the local electrogram (ABL d) shows low-amplitude fractionated potentials. (b) RF delivery results in arrhythmia termination.

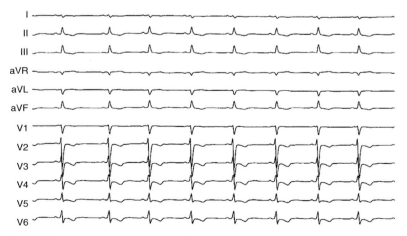

Figure 19.6 A 12-lead ECG after restoration of sinus rhythm.

CHAPTER 20

Recurrent atrial flutter after isthmus ablation

David Callans, MD, FACC, FHRS

Clinical vignette

A 64-year-old man with hypertension but no structural heart disease had typical counterclockwise atrial flutter, and underwent isthmus ablation. Bidirectional block was demonstrated at the end of the procedure. He was well for 2 weeks, but then developed rapid palpitations and near syncope. Paramedics recorded the following strips on arrival (Figure 20.1) and treated the patient with cardioversion.

Because of a clinical suspicion of recurrent atrial flutter with 1:1 conduction, an electrophysiology (EP) study was performed.

Electrophysiology study and ablation

Halo-type multielectrode catheter recordings during coronary sinus (CS) pacing were originally interpreted as showing persistent isthmus block (CS stim – RA low = 93) (Figure 20.2). However, EnSite Array mapping demonstrated conduction through a small gap in the isthmus line (Figure 20.3). Atrial flutter was induced, and concealed entrainment was demonstrated from the isthmus (Figure 20.4). Two radiofrequency lesions were delivered to the gap in the isthmus line, leading to termination of atrial flutter. Afterward, EnSite Array mapping during CS pacing demonstrated isthmus block, with double potentials in unipolar recordings along the ablation line (Figure 20.5). This case demonstrates the difficulties with the definition of isthmus conduction block. No matter how long the conduction time between the CS and the low lateral RA measures, it is difficult to diagnose block as opposed to slow persistent conduction without many recordings close to the ablation line. This can be done with the array system, as in this case, or with careful retracing of the line with the mapping catheter.

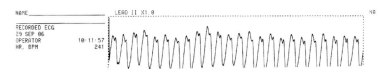

Figure 20.1 Wide complex tachycardia recorded by paramedics.

Electroanatomical Mapping, 1st edition. Edited by
A. Al-Ahmad, D. Callans, H. Hsia and A. Natale.
© 2008 Blackwell Publishing, ISBN: 9781405157025.

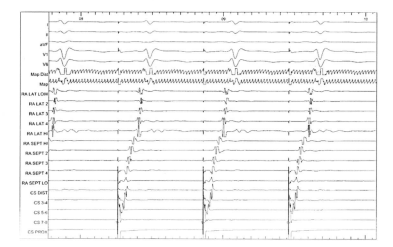

Figure 20.2 Halo catheter recording with pacing from the coronary sinus.

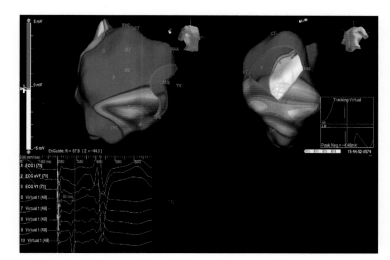

Figure 20.3 EnSite Array map showing conduction through the cavotricuspid isthmus.

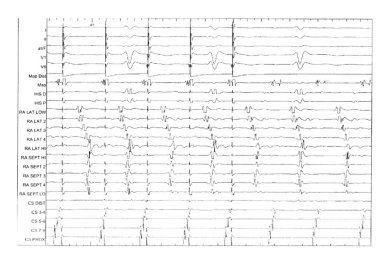

Figure 20.4 Induced atrial flutter with concealed entrainment from the isthmus.

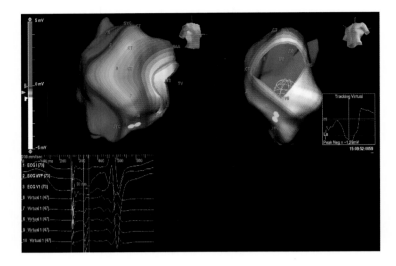

Figure 20.5   EnSite Array map demonstrating complete isthmus block. See the double potentials on the virtual recording.

CHAPTER 21

Scar-based reentrant atrial tachycardia in a patient with congenital heart disease

Ricarrdo Capato, MD

Clinical vignette

A 31-year-old woman with a history of congenital heart disease became symptomatic with palpitations and, subsequently, developed congestive heart failure. Her heart disease consisted of single ventricle associated with pulmonary atresia, atrial right isomerism, and common AV valve. The patient underwent Waterson intervention early after birth and modified Fontan intervention at the age of 6. She recently developed palpitations associated with

heart failure, the 12-lead EKG documented a regular atrial tachycardia (Figure 21.1). She had previously undergone two successful electrical cardioversions, but in both cases experienced early recurrence despite therapy with sotalol and, subsequently, amiodarone. A cardiac catheterization demonstrated good anatomical and functional results from previous cardiac surgery and no need for further cardiac interventions. She was then referred to our electrophysiology (EP) lab for electrophysiological study and catheter ablation of the atrial tachycardia.

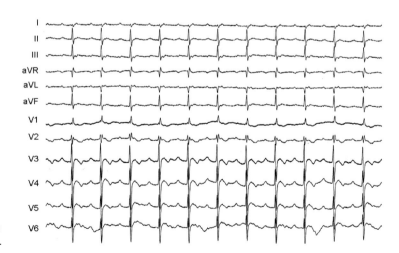

Figure 21.1 Atrial tachycardia at 150 bpm, with 2:1 AV conduction.

Electroanatomical Mapping, 1st edition. Edited by
A. Al-Ahmad, D. Callans, H. Hsia and A. Natale.
© 2008 Blackwell Publishing, ISBN: 9781405157025.

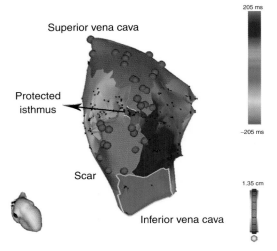

205 ms

−205 ms

1.35 cm

Figure 21.2   Right anterior oblique projection showing the three-dimensional reconstructed CARTO™ map during atrial tachycardia. Note the protected isthmus within two large areas of scar along the posterior-lateral right atrial wall.

Electrophysiology study and ablation

Electroanatomical mapping was performed using a three-dimensional CARTO™ map. A macroreentrant circuit was identified in the right atrium with two large areas of scar tissue along the posterior-lateral wall surrounding a protected isthmus of viable tissue in which slow conduction was found (Figure 21.2). Voltage mapping in the right atrium showed low-amplitude potentials widely distributed in the entire chamber (Figure 21.3). Radiofrequency pulse delivery within the protected isthmus resulted in immediate termination of the clinical arrhythmia (Figure 21.3), which was not re-inducible thereafter.

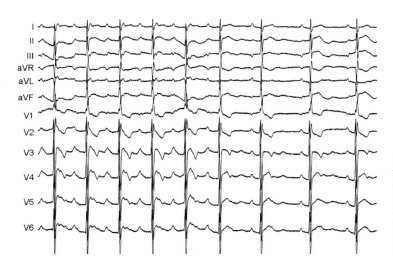

Figure 21.3   A few seconds after the onset of radiofrequency delivery within the protected isthmus, termination of atrial arrhythmia is observed with restoration of an atrial escape rhythm at 60 bpm, exhibiting a negative P wave in lead III.

CHAPTER 22

A case of post-MAZE atrial flutter

Tamer S. Fahmy, MD, *& Andrea Natale,* MD

Clinical vignette

The patient is a 64-year-old male who presents with a past medical history significant for chronic atrial fibrillation (CAF) and valvular heart disease. In the past 7 years, he has had multiple congestive heart hospitalizations exacerbated by atrial fibrillation. His past cardiac surgical history is significant for aortic valve replacement, followed 10 years later by mitral and tricuspid valve repair and concomitant MAZE procedure. However, he is still suffering from recurrent episodes of AF and flutter, which is refractory to more than one antiarrhythmic drug (tikosyn and amiodarone). He was considered for ablation.

His ECG during tachycardia revealed atrial flutter with variable ventricular response, and positive flutter waves in the inferior leads consistent with atypical atrial flutter (Figure 22.1a). Another ECG performed while the patient was in AF is shown in Figure 22.1b. His echocardiography revealed biatrial enlargement and moderate tricuspid regurgitation.

Electrophysiology study and ablation

The patient entered the electrophysiology (EP) lab in atrial flutter (Figures 22.2 and 22.3). Given the patient's history of a prior maze procedure, ECG showing atypical flutter, the LA was mapped first.

An activation map of the LA revealed a radial activation pattern, with the earliest activation found at the septum (Figure 22.4). At this point, the possibilities were focal tachycardia from the septum or a right-sided tachycardia with the earliest breakthrough at the septum. Given the fact that the LA map could not account for the whole cycle length, the RA was subsequently mapped.

Mapping of the RA revealed a line of double potentials at the posterolateral RA wall. This line of block was likely to be at the site of the surgical scar created to enter the RA. The flutter circuit propagates around the scar (Figure 22.5). The double potentials were traced along the line, and a region was found where both potentials were very close, indicating the gap in the line of block. Few lesions at the area of close double potentials terminated the tachycardia with no further induction (Figure 22.6a and b).

Going back to the LA to check the pulmonary veins (PVs), a Lasso catheter was introduced and revealed recovery of potentials from the four PVs, which has been missed with the 4-mm Navistar catheter during the initial mapping. This scar area appeared to cover the whole antrum as seen on the intracardiac echo (Figure 22.7). The four veins were re-isolated, and finally a cavotricuspid isthmus (CTI) line was drawn, after differential pacing revealed persistence of conduction along the CTI.

Of interest, the CARTO™ map showed two separate left PV ostia and it was unable to depict the large left common ostium seen on the echo (Figure 22.7).

Electroanatomical Mapping, 1st edition. Edited by A. Al-Ahmad, D. Callans, H. Hsia and A. Natale.
© 2008 Blackwell Publishing, ISBN: 9781405157025.

(a)

(b)

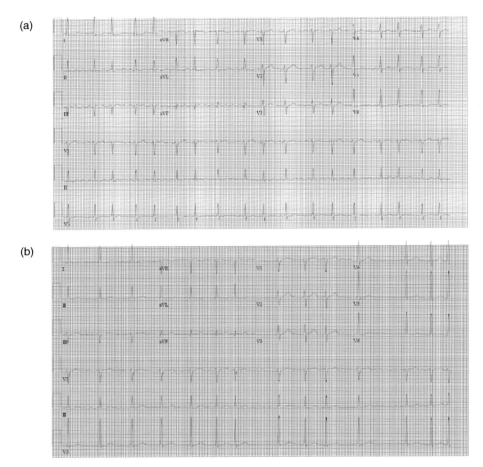

Figure 22.1 Twelve-lead surface ECGs of the patient prior to the ablation procedure. Panel a shows the atrial flutter with variable ventricular response. The flutter waves (250 ms) appear to be positive in the inferior leads as well as V1, consistent with atypical flutter. Panel b shows another episode of AF.

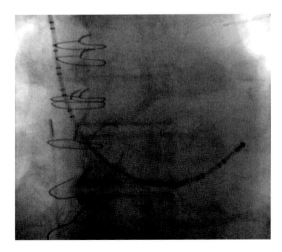

Figure 22.2 Fluoroscopic image in left anterior oblique (LAO) view (30°) showing the mitral and tricuspid valve rings. A duo-decapolar coronary sinus catheter is in place, and the intracardiac echo probe is seen in the RA.

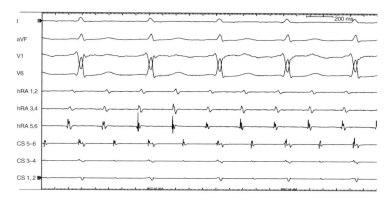

Figure 22.3   From top to bottom, three surface ECG leads followed by intracardiac recording along the lateral wall of the high right atrium (HRA 1–6) and finally the coronary sinus (CS 1–6). Regular tachycardia with A-A cycle length of 250 ms is shown where the activation sequence appears from low to high along the lateral wall. This also seems to precede the CS activation.

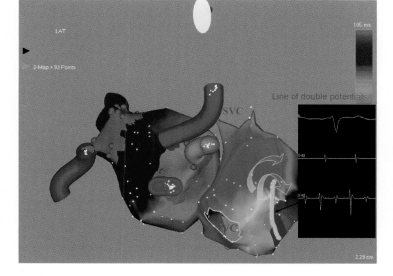

Figure 22.4   An electroanatomical activation map of the LA, constructed during atrial flutter. The gray areas around the pulmonary indicate scar areas as mapped by the Navistar catheter. The map shows a radial activation pattern with the earliest activation site at the septum. Note that based on the CARTO™ map the patient seems to have two separate left PV ostia.

Figure 22.5   Activation map of both atria in right posterior oblique (RPO) view. A line of double potentials is seen on the right atrial posterolateral wall. This line of block was assumed to represent the operative scar created to enter the right atrium. The map shows a circular activation pattern rotating around the line of block, with further spreading of activation to both atria.

(a)

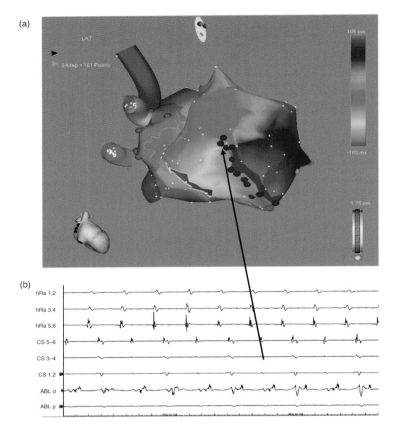

(b)

Figure 22.6 Panel A shows the activation map of both atria with the ablation line created at the gap on the line of double potentials. Panel B shows the intracardiac recording with the ablation catheter placed at the successful site. As shown, the distance between the double potentials on the ablation catheter seems very small, indicating a possible gap in the line. Ablation in this area terminated the tachycardia.

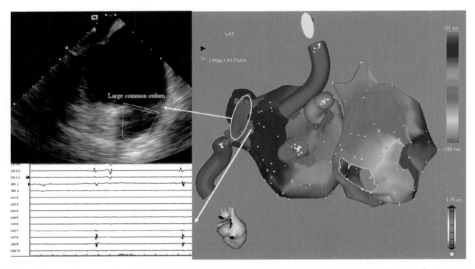

Figure 22.7 A large antrum with a large common ostium was mapped as a scar by a 4-mm Navistar catheter. Mapping with the Lasso catheter at the same location revealed persistence of electrical connection within the PVs and the presence of potentials that have been missed with the 4-mm catheter. In addition, note that the CARTO™ map is unable to detect the presence of the large common ostium as shown on echo.

CHAPTER 23

A case of atypical atrial flutter

Tamer Fahmy, MD, *Dimpi Patel,* MD, *& Andrea Natale,* MD

Clinical vignette

The patient is a 54-year-old male with a past medical history significant for chronic atrial flutter (AFL), hypertension, hyperlipidemia, and diabetes mellitus.

In 2004, he had a previous ablation for atypical flutter that was performed at an outside institution. This was unsuccessful. Three months after the ablation he continued to experience palpitations, and appeared to be in persistent AFL. His ECG during tachycardia revealed AFL with positive flutter waves in V1 and isoelectric in the inferior leads (rate 250 ms) (Figure 23.1). In the past, he had been electrically cardioverted and was successfully maintained on antiarrhythmic medications. However, recently antiarrhythmic medications were not able to control his AFL. Therefore, he was considered for repeat radiofrequency ablation.

Electrophysiology study and ablation

The patient was in AFL when he arrived in the electrophysiology (EP) lab. As his ECG was not consistent with typical AFL, and more consistent with a left-sided AFL, the LA was mapped first. An electroanatomical activation map was performed of the LA, which accounted for the whole cycle length of the tachycardia. The activation map showed a macroreentrant circuit which propagated around the right pulmonary veins and the scar around the veins of unknown origin (Figure 23.2). At the roof anterior to the right pulmonary veins, there was

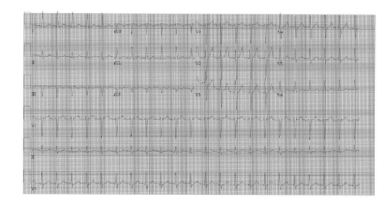

Figure 23.1 Twelve-lead ECG during tachycardia. The flutter waves (250 ms) appear to be isoelectric in the inferior leads and positive in lead V1.

Electroanatomical Mapping, 1st edition. Edited by
A. Al-Ahmad, D. Callans, H. Hsia and A. Natale.
© 2008 Blackwell Publishing, ISBN: 9781405157025.

an area showing double and fractionated potentials; this area was thought to encompass the critical isthmus. Ablation lesions at that location failed to terminate the tachycardia (Figure 23.3). At this point the whole activation map was revised, and another relatively early area was found just between the mitral valve and the atrial appendage, which did not fit with the activation sequence as viewed on the isochronal and propagation maps (Figures 23.4 and 23.5). Although the window of interest was set to accommodate only one cycle, there were double and fractionated electrograms (EGMs) of long duration that created confusion during point acquisition. These points were revised and re-annotated to the other EGM within the window of interest (Figure 23.6). This resulted in a complete change of the flutter circuit, which now appeared to circulate around the mitral valve and converge passively anteriorly and posteriorly to the right pulmonary veins, to the same area initially thought to encompass the circuit (Figures 23.7 and 23.8). After the left isthmus line failed to terminate the tachycardia, an anterior line was created to the mitral annulus that successfully terminated the tachycardia. The tachycardia could not be re-induced.

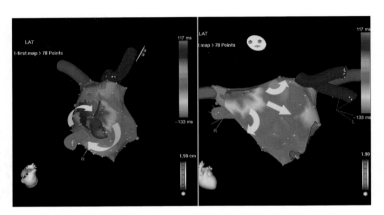

Figure 23.2 Initial activation map during tachycardia. Right panel (anteroposterior [AP] cranial) shows earliest activation anterior to the right superior pulmonary vein (RSPV) and the white arrows shows the activation sequence. The left panel (right lateral cranial) reveals a circular activation pattern, rotating around the right pulmonary veins and the surrounding scar of unknown origin.

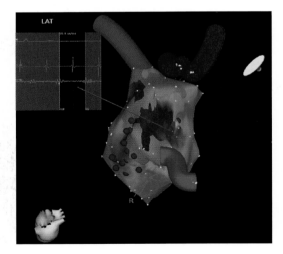

Figure 23.3 Ablation lesions created at the areas showing fractionation and double potentials. These lesions could not terminate the tachycardia.

Figure 23.4 By revising the activation map, a seven-color isochronal map of the activation wave front was created which depicts an area of early activation below the left superior pulmonary vein (LSVP), which does not fit with the sequence of activation, which seemed to have been overlooked in the normal view (Figure 23.2, right panel).

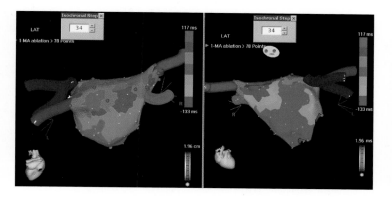

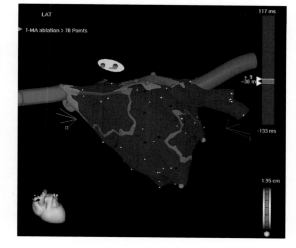

Figure 23.5 Propagation map for the initial activation sequence, showing the propagating wave front moving down and to the left along the anterior wall. However, there is another propagating wave front moving in the opposite direction. Changing the annotation on the lower point to the late EGM has not solved the problem as it was much later than the latest activation, and changed the map to radial activation (focal) rather than a circular one.

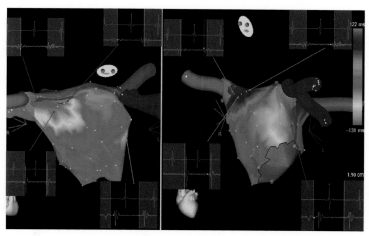

Figure 23.6 Changes in annotation. The left panel (AP cranial) shows the initial activation map with the electrograms acquired and annotated selected at the areas of interest. The window of interest has been set at 90% of the tachycardia cycle length. Note the fractionated and double potentials recorded from the area where early meet late at which the initial ablation was performed. The right panel (left anterior oblique, LAO) shows the change in the activation map after changing the annotation of the EGMs at some of the areas of interest. The activation sequence appears to circulate around the mitral valve.

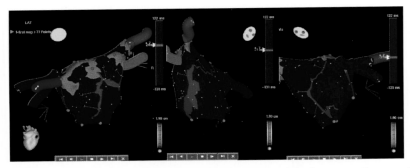

Figure 23.7   Propagation map of the readjusted activation map. From right to left, the propagating wave front seems to be moving in a counterclockwise direction around the mitral valve, and passively encircling the right pulmonary veins which caused confusion with the initial map.

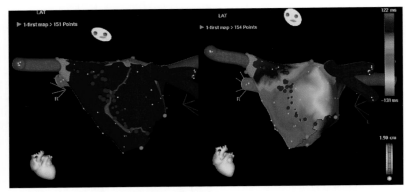

Figure 23.8   Activation (right) and propagation maps (left) showing the anterior ablation line, going down to the mitral valve and interrupting the active tachycardia circuit.

CHAPTER 24

Spontaneous scar-based atypical and typical AFL

Greg Feld, MD

Clinical vignette

The patient is a self-referred, 27-year-old female, with a history of atrial flutter (AFL), who underwent attempted AFL ablation at another hospital, resulting in inadvertent AV node ablation. A dual-chamber pacemaker was therefore implanted. This was followed by an atrial lead revision for lead dislodgement. The patient now presents with continued symptoms including dizziness, near syncope, palpitations, chest pain, and shortness of breath. The patient had a normal physical examination. Further evaluation at our institution revealed atrial lead malfunction with a high pacing threshold greater than 5 V and atrial undersensing. The patient also had complete AV block.

Further pacemaker interrogation revealed recurrent paroxysmal AFL (Figure 24.1). An atrial lead extraction was performed with atrial lead replacement. The patient was treated temporarily with flecainide and a beta-blocker with marked improvement of symptoms. The flecainide was subsequently discontinued and the patient underwent electrophysiology (EP) study and ablation of two AFLs. At the 2-year follow-up, the patient has had no further AFL.

Electrophysiology study and ablation

Surface ECG and endocardial tracing show an atypical AFL, the coronary sinus (CS) activation

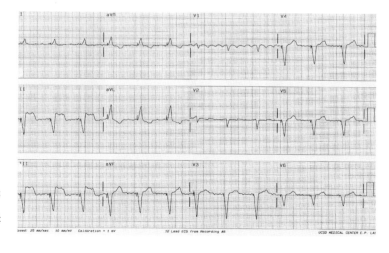

Figure 24.1 A 12-lead ECG showing AFL, cycle length 230 ms, AV block, and ventricular pacing. The F wave is positive in lead I, negative in V1, and flat or biphasic in all other leads, suggesting a probable right atrial origin but not a typical AFL.

Electroanatomical Mapping, 1st edition. Edited by
A. Al-Ahmad, D. Callans, H. Hsia and A. Natale.
© 2008 Blackwell Publishing, ISBN: 9781405157025.

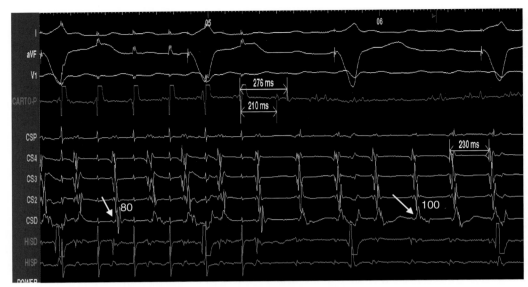

Figure 24.2   Surface ECG and endocardial tracings, showing an atypical AFL, but with proximal to distal CS activation sequence, suggesting right atrial origin. There was AV block with ventricular pacing. Pacing from the cavotricuspid isthmus (CTI) demonstrated overt entrainment, suggesting that the CTI was not within circuit. Note the different conduction time from the stimulus artifact (CARTO-P) in the CTI to the proximal coronary sinus (proximal CS) of 80 ms, compared to the conduction time from the local electrogram in the CTI (CARTO-P) to the proximal CS of 100 ms.

sequence suggests a right atrial origin. Pacing from the cavotricuspid isthmus (CTI) demonstrated overt entrainment, suggesting that the CTI was not within the circuit (Figure 24.2). An electroanatomical activation map demonstrated a lower loop tachycardia rotating counterclockwise around the inferior vena cava, utilizing the scar isthmus as an area of slow conduction. Ablation was performed at the scar isthmus to eliminate transverse conduction through scar, resulting in complete block along the scar zone. Following ablation, AFL was sustained, but the cycle length actually shortened from 230 ms to 216 ms, and there was a change in the 12-lead ECG F-wave morphology and endocardial activation pattern (Figure 24.3). The CS activation sequence still suggests a right atrial origin (Figure 24.4). Surface ECG lead F-wave morphology (inverted in aVF and V1) is now suggestive of typical AFL (Figure 24.5). Pacing from the CTI demonstrating concealed entrainment, confirming typical CTI isthmus dependent AFL. Ablation in the CTI resulted in the elimination of AFL and resumption of normal sinus rhythm with ventricular pacing (Figures 24.6 and 24.7).

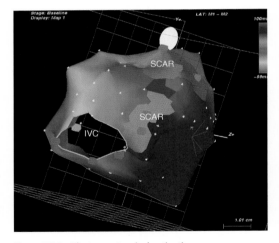

Figure 24.3   Electroanatomical activation map demonstrating a lower loop tachycardia rotating counterclockwise around the inferior vena cava, utilizing the scar isthmus as an area of slow conduction. Ablation was performed at the scar isthmus to eliminate transverse conduction through scar, resulting in complete block along the scar zone. Following ablation, AFL was sustained, but the cycle length actually shortened from 230 ms to 216 ms, and there was a change in the 12-lead ECG F-wave morphology and endocardial activation pattern. IVC = inferior vena cava.

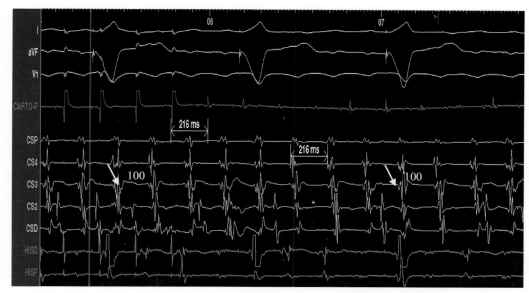

Figure 24.4 Surface ECG and endocardial tracings during persistent AFL following ablation of posterior scar isthmus. Note the change in cycle length to from 230 to 216 ms, but with persistent proximal to distal CS activation sequence suggesting a right atrial origin. Note the change surface ECG lead F-wave morphology (inverted in aVF and V1) suggestive of typical AFL. Pacing from the CTI demonstrating concealed entrainment, confirming typical CTI isthmus dependent AFL. Note the equivalent first postpacing interval and AFL cycle length, and the equivalent stimulus to coronary sinus electrogram (proximal CS) interval and pacing site electrogram (CARTO-P) to proximal CS electrogram interval.

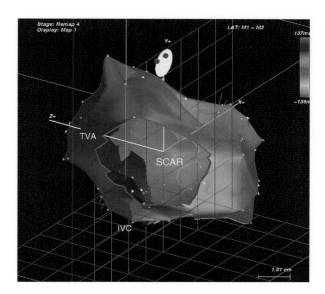

Figure 24.5 Electroanatomical activation map demonstrating typical (counterclockwise) AFL around the tricuspid valve annulus, through the CTI, and around the posterior right atrial scar. IVC = inferior vena cava; TVA = tricuspid valve annulus

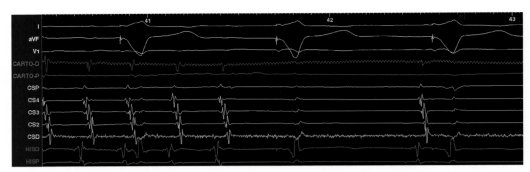

Figure 24.6 Surface ECG and endocardial tracings during ablation of the CTI. Note termination of typical AFL during CTI ablation, with subsequent restoration of AV sequential pacing (atrial sensing and ventricular pacing).

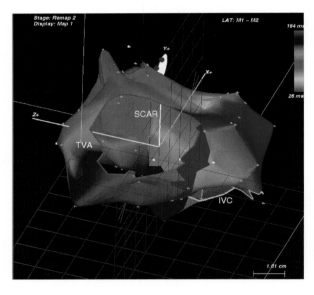

Figure 24.7 Electroanatomical activation map demonstrating medial to lateral CTI block during pacing from the proximal coronary sinus following CTI ablation. Lateral to medial CTI block was also demonstrated (not shown) during pacing from the low lateral right atrium (bidirectional CTI block). IVC = inferior vena cava; TVA = tricuspid valve annulus

CHAPTER 25

Left atrial flutter after pulmonary vein isolation

Richard Hongo, MD *& Andrea Natale,* MD, FACC, FHRS

Clinical vignette

A 61-year-old man presented with a persistent atrial arrhythmia after two previous pulmonary vein isolation ablations for atrial fibrillation. A third electrophysiology (EP) study had just been completed at another institution, but ablation had not been performed after the arrhythmia was interpreted to be a para-hisian atrial tachycardia. The heart rate during the atrial arrhythmia was 105 bpm. P waves on the 12-lead ECG (Figure 25.1) were relatively narrow and occurred equidistant from the preceding and following R waves.

Electrophysiology study and ablation

A fourth EP study was performed and intracardiac electrograms revealed an atrial arrhythmia twice the ventricular rate with a tachycardia cycle length of 280 ms. A three-dimensional electroanatomic (CARTO™ system; Biosense Webster) map of the right atrium (RA) demonstrated earliest activation originating from a relatively wide region along the septum (Figure 25.2). The entire RA activation, however, only accounted for 66 ms of the tachycardia cycle length and preceded the distal coronary

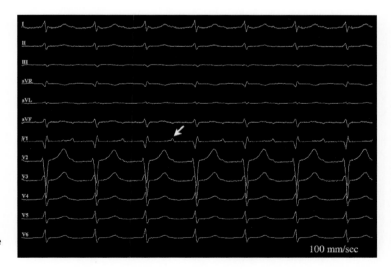

Figure 25.1 A 12-lead ECG of the atrial flutter. Note the flutter wave (arrow).

100 mm/sec

Electroanatomical Mapping, 1st edition. Edited by
A. Al-Ahmad, D. Callans, H. Hsia and A. Natale.
© 2008 Blackwell Publishing, ISBN: 9781405157025.

sinus reference activation by over 50 ms. This observation meant that atrial activation had to originate from the left atrium (LA). A trans-septal puncture was performed and a three-dimensional electroanatomic map of the LA was created (Figure 25.3). Activation around a scar that was anterior to the right upper pulmonary vein (RUPV) spanned the entire tachycardia cycle length (276 ms), suggesting that the atrial arrhythmia was in fact atrial flutter. An isthmus was identified between this scar and the RUPV. The electrogram at this isthmus demonstrated low-amplitude fractionated signal that spanned nearly one-fourth of the flutter cycle length, and included a single higher-amplitude discrete potential (Figure 25.4). Radiofrequency ablation at this site resulted in immediate termination of the atrial flutter. The patient has maintained sinus rhythm following this fourth procedure.

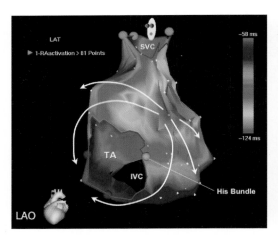

Figure 25.2 CARTO™ map of the right atrium. Note the wide area of early activation and that despite a comprehensive anatomical map – only 66 ms of the tachycardia cycle length have been accounted for in this map.

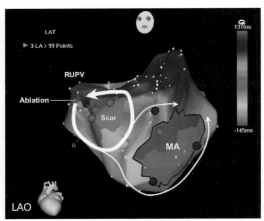

Figure 25.3 Left atrial CARTO™ activation map showing the atrial flutter circuit and the area of ablation. Note that in this map 276 ms of the tachycardia cycle length is accounted for.

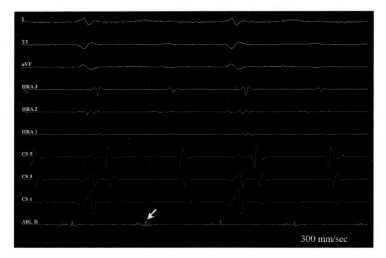

Figure 25.4 Ablation at this site terminated the atrial flutter. Note the discrete potential (arrow).

26 CHAPTER 26

Scar-based reentrant atrial tachycardia

Henry Hsia, MD

Clinical vignette

The patient is a 58-year-old man with a history of atrial septal defect repair and mitral valve repair. He had various postoperative tachycardias and underwent a right atrial flutter ablation.

The patient developed recurrent atrial arrhythmias that were refractory to amiodarone (Figure 26.1). He is referred for a repeat catheter ablation.

A cardiac catheterization demonstrated only minimal coronary luminal irregularities. An echocardiogram showed an ejection fraction of 45% with trace aortic and mitral regurgitations. Mild-to-moderate tricuspid regurgitation was present with moderate pulmonary hypertension.

Electrophysiology study and ablation

Electroanatomical mapping showed two large posterior right atrial scars. Activation and entrainment mapping revealed a macroreentry circuit (Figure 26.2). Using the surface P waves as a reference, a clockwise reentry was demonstrated (atrial tachycardia #1). The wave front propagates around the superior scar, traverse across the "isthmus" between the scars (Figure 26.3).

A second tachycardia was induced (atrial tachycardia #2). Using the earliest intracardiac activation (halo 4) a reference, a counterclockwise reentry was demonstrated. The wave front propagates

#1: Atrial tachycardia: cycle length of ~400 ms

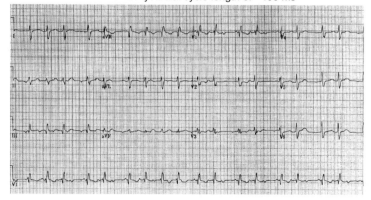

Figure 26.1 Atypical atrial flutter. The "flutter" waves were relatively narrow, lacked the positive terminal forces, and had long isoelectric intervals.

Electroanatomical Mapping, 1st edition. Edited by A. Al-Ahmad, D. Callans, H. Hsia and A. Natale. © 2008 Blackwell Publishing, ISBN: 9781405157025.

around the superior scar in a reversed direction through the "isthmus" (Figure 26.4).

Multicomponent electrograms were recorded at the "isthmus" between the scars. Radiofrequency energy delivery at sites with "fused" potentials successfully terminated the tachycardias (Figure 26.5). Linear ablation was performed to connect the scars and transect the isthmus.

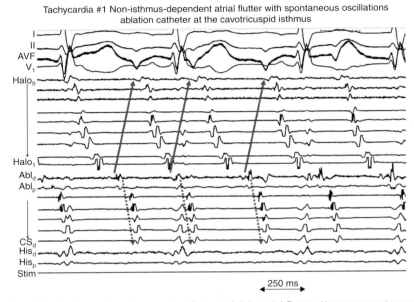

Figure 26.2 The atrial activation pattern is suggestive of a typical right atrial flutter. However, spontaneous heart rate variations demonstrated the oscillation of the ablation catheter recordings at the cavotricuspid isthmus preceded the oscillations of the coronary sinus (CS) and the lateral right atrial recordings (halo), and is not dependent of the counterclockwise activation of the halo. The tachycardia also cannot be entrained at the isthmus site.

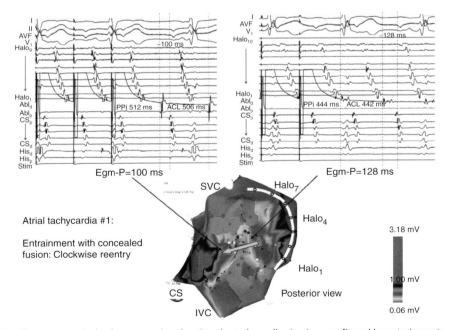

Figure 26.3 Electroanatomical voltage mapping showing the tachycardia circuit as confirmed by entrainment.

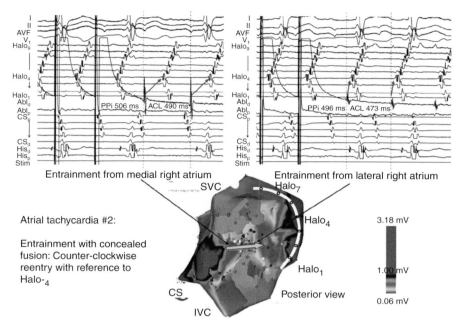

Figure 26.4   Entrainment and mapping of the second atrial flutter that utilizes the same isthmus.

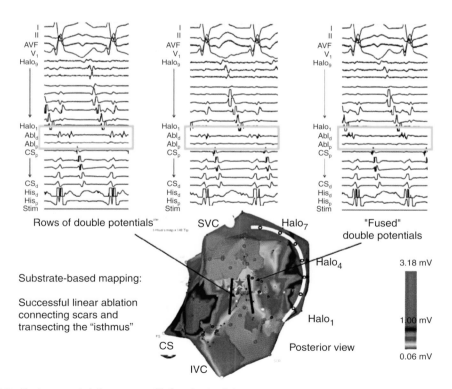

Figure 26.5   Electrograms in isthmus area with fused potentials.

CHAPTER 27

Atypical atrial flutter following circumferential left atrial ablation

James David Allred, MD *Harish Doppalapudi,* MD &
G. Neal Kay, MD

Clinical vignette

The patient is a 68-year-old male with recurrent symptomatic atrial flutter presents for catheter ablation. He underwent pulmonary vein isolation and cavotricuspid isthmus (CTI) ablation 3 months earlier for atrial fibrillation and counterclockwise, isthmus-dependent atrial flutter. During the procedure, he developed left atrial flutter consistent with mitral annular reentry and also underwent mitral isthmus ablation with successful termination of the flutter. Over the next 3 months he developed incessant palpitations and was found to have atrial flutter on ECG (Figure 27.1).

Electrophysiology study and ablation

Atrial flutter around the mitral valve annulus can occur despite an initial ECG that could be confused with CTI-dependent atrial flutter. Transient entrainment from the region between the mitral valve annulus and the left inferior pulmonary vein demonstrated a postpacing interval equal to the tachycardia cycle length, proving that this region was involved within the reentrant circuit (Figures 27.2 and 27.3). Following wide area circumferential pulmonary vein isolation there is an increased risk of macroreentrant left atrial tachycardias. The ECG

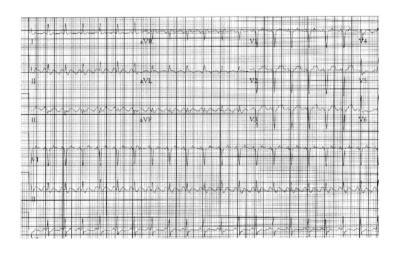

Figure 27.1 The 12-lead ECG shows atrial flutter with 2:1 conduction. The atrial flutter waves are upright in V1 with a sawtooth pattern in II, III, and aVF. The atrial cycle length is 200 ms. In the inferior leads, the flutter waves have a biphasic morphology with an initial negative followed by positive polarity.

Electroanatomical Mapping, 1st edition. Edited by
A. Al-Ahmad, D. Callans, H. Hsia and A. Natale.
© 2008 Blackwell Publishing, ISBN: 9781405157025.

pattern of atrial flutter may be misleading such that left atrial flutters may mimic right atrial flutter and CTI-dependent atrial flutters may mimic left atrial flutters. Catheter ablation of circum-mitral annular left atrial flutter often requires ablation of the coronary sinus musculature (Figures 27.4 and 27.5).

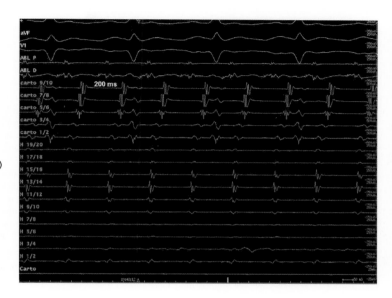

Figure 27.2 Surface electrocardiographic leads I, aVF, and V1 are recorded simultaneously with bipolar intracardiac electrograms in the left atrium proximal (ABL P) and distal (ABL D) electrode pairs, coronary sinus proximal (CARTO 9/10) through distal (CARTO 1/2) electrode pairs with a 20-pole Lasso circular catheter (H1/2 through 19/20) in the roof of the left atrium. Note that the atrial cycle length is 200 ms with distal to proximal activation in the coronary sinus.

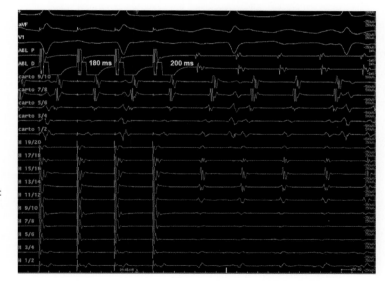

Figure 27.3 Rapid atrial pacing from the left atrial catheter positioned between the left inferior pulmonary vein and the mitral annulus at a cycle length of 180 ms. Following the last pacing stimulus, the postpacing interval at the (ABL D) electrogram measured 200 ms, identical to the atrial flutter cycle length of 200 ms. Thus, this left atrial isthmus is proven to be located within the reentrant circuit.

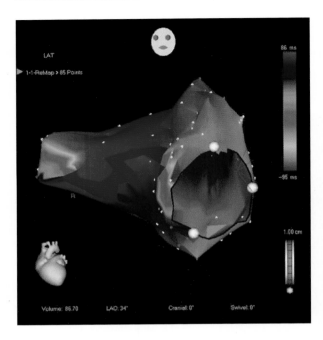

Figure 27.4 CARTO™ local activation map of the left atrium as viewed from the left anterior oblique projection with caudal angulation. The activation pattern demonstrates clockwise rotation around the mitral valve annulus. The activation time around the mitral valve annulus accounts for over 90% of the cycle length of the circuit. Catheter ablation between the mitral valve annulus and the left inferior pulmonary vein slowed but failed to terminate the left atrial flutter. Termination was achieved with ablation within the mid-portion of the coronary sinus.

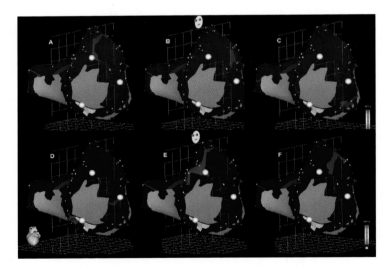

Figure 27.5 Propagation map of circum-mitral annulus left atrial flutter. There is progressive activation in a clockwise pattern (A–F).

CHAPTER 28

Scar-related intraatrial reentrant tachycardia

Kevin Makati, MD *& N. A. Mark Estes III,* MD

Clinical vignette

A 53-year-old male presented with symptomatic supraventricular tachycardia. His past medical history is significant for congenital aortic stenosis corrected with a Ross procedure 15 years prior to presentation. Two years prior to presentation, the patient developed symptomatic typical atrial flutter. Rate suppressive medications were poorly tolerated and he underwent a successful radiofrequency (RF) ablation of the cavotricuspid isthmus. Shortly after, the patient had recurrence of atrial flutter; however, the second tachycardia appeared atypical on the basis of morphology on the surface tracing (Figure 28.1).

Electrophysiology study and ablation

Electrograms from the coronary sinus catheter seemed to be consistent with a right-sided tachycardia (Figure 28.2). An electroanatomical activation map of the right atrium revealed an area of scar in the lateral right atrium (Figure 28.3). The wave front appeared to be using the scar as a fixed boarder of the circuit. Entrainment mapping demonstrated concealed entrainment and a perfect postpacing interval (Figure 28.4). Ablation between the scar and the inferior vena cava resulted in elimination of the atrial flutter (Figures 28.5 and 28.6). Non-cavotricuspid-isthmus-dependent intraatrial

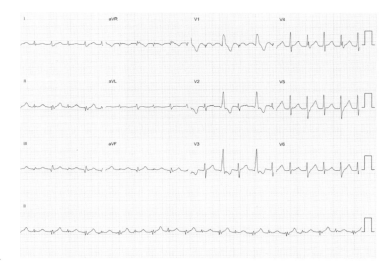

Figure 28.1 A 12-lead electrocardiogram shows an atrial flutter.

Electroanatomical Mapping, 1st edition. Edited by
A. Al-Ahmad, D. Callans, H. Hsia and A. Natale.
© 2008 Blackwell Publishing, ISBN: 9781405157025.

reentrant tachycardia is commonly seen in patients with right atrial incisional scars created during cardiac surgery for retrograde cardioplegia infusion via the coronary sinus. The flutter circuit may involve any area of functional scar in the atrium and ranges from simple circuits to complex circuits that travel in a figure of eight pattern. Interruption of the tachycardia circuit is performed by ablation in the critical isthmus that can be defined by areas of scar or anatomical boarders.

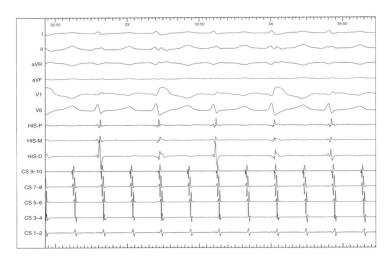

Figure 28.2 The intracardiac tracing shows an intraatrial reentrant tachycardia with earliest atrial activation at coronary sinus bipole pair 9 and 10.

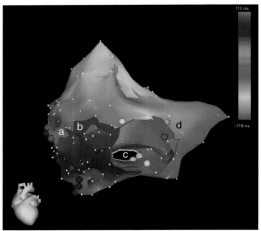

Figure 28.3 An electroanatomic map using CARTO™ is constructed of the right atrium in the left anterior oblique projection while in the tachycardia. An early wave front, shown in orange, travels between an area of scar (a) marked in gray, and the tricuspid annulus (d) and meets an area of late activation in purple at the area (b) inferior vena cava (IVC) (c).

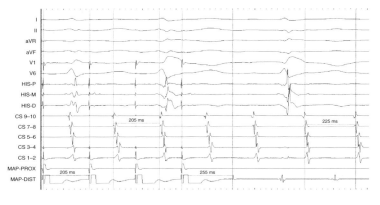

Figure 28.4 Entrainment of the tachycardia is performed at a rate that is 20 ms faster than the cycle length of the tachycardia (225 ms). The postpacing interval (PPI) is 225 ms.

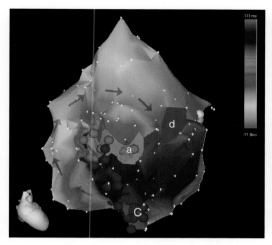

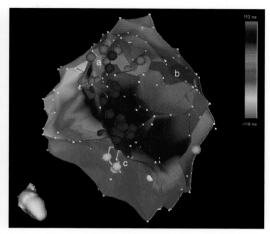

Figure 28.5 Electroanatomic map of the tachycardia in the right anterior oblique projection showing the intraatrial reentrant tachycardia revolve around the area of scar (a) in the anterolateral right atrium. The earliest wave front meets the latest wave front at the area in red (b). Using RF ablation, a line connecting the area of scar and the inferior vena cava is created (c).

Figure 28.6 Electroanatomic map of the tachycardia in the right anterior oblique projection with caudal angulation during the intraatrial reentrant tachycardia revolving around an area of scar (a). A red line (b) shows where the earliest area of activation meets the latest. Using RF ablation, a line is created between the area of scar and the inferior vena cava (c).

CHAPTER 29

Electroanatomic mapping for atrial flutter

Pirooz Mofrad, MD *& Amin Al-Ahmad,* MD

Clinical vignette

A 41-year-old male with no significant past medical history was referred with frequent symptomatic paroxysms of atrial flutter despite treatment with antiarrhythmic medications. A 12-lead EKG (Figure 29.1) was consistent with typical isthmus-dependent counterclockwise atrial flutter.

Electrophysiology study and ablation

The patient underwent a diagnostic electrophysiology study with inducible typical right atrial flutter that was successfully entrained from the cavotricuspid isthmus with a postpacing interval approximating the tachycardia cycle length. Catheter mapping and ablation using the CARTO™ three-dimensional mapping system was performed (Figure 29.2). Bidirectional conduction block was achieved with the delivery of linear lesions along the cavotricuspid isthmus (Figure 29.3).

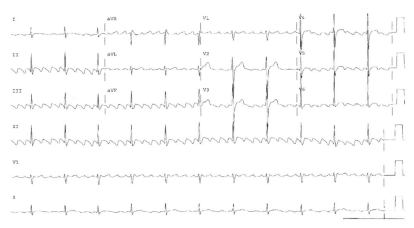

Figure 29.1 A 12-lead EKG of the patient with typical isthmus-dependent right atrial flutter.

Electroanatomical Mapping, 1st edition. Edited by
A. Al-Ahmad, D. Callans, H. Hsia and A. Natale.
© 2008 Blackwell Publishing, ISBN: 9781405157025.

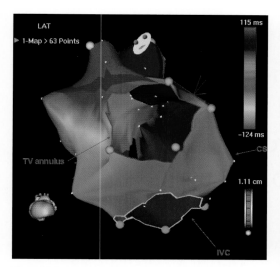

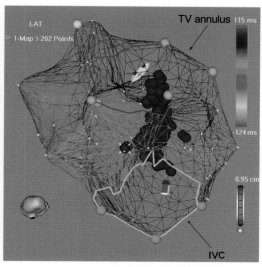

Figure 29.2 Activation map: Superiorly directed lateral view of the right atrial activation map during typical right atrial isthmus-dependent flutter with "early meets late" activation pattern. The cavotricuspid isthmus is clearly delineated and was the target for linear radiofrequency ablation lesions. TV refers to tricuspid valve, CS refers to coronary sinus os, and IVC refers to inferior vena cava.

Figure 29.3 Superiorly directed lateral view of the Mesh map consisting of linear ablation lesions directed to the cavotricuspid isthmus that terminated the atrial flutter with noninducibility and evidence of bidirectional block with pacing from the lower lateral and septal walls of the right atrium.

CHAPTER 30

Electroanatomical mapping for incessant small macroreentrant left atrial tachycardia following catheter ablation of atrial fibrillation

Hiroshi Nakagawa, MD, PhD *& Warren M. Jackman,* MD

Clinical vignette

A 45-year-old woman with a history of surgical closure of an atrial septal defect at age 5 was evaluated for atrial tachycardia (AT). She had episodes of palpitations for the past 15 years despite medical therapy. She underwent three prior catheter ablation procedures: (1) ablation of typical right atrial flutter (AFL) in May 2002; (2) segmental isolation of the pulmonary veins (PVs) and repeat ablation of typical AFL in October 2002; and (3) wide circumferential PV ablation and left atrial linear ablation along the mitral isthmus and between the left and right circumferential PV ablation lines (without confirmation of complete PV isolation or block across left atrial lines) in March 2003. One month after the third ablation procedure, she developed incessant atrial tachycardia (AT) resistant to five antiarrhythmic medications (including amiodarone) (Figure 30.1). She was referred to our center for catheter ablation of the incessant AT in April 2004.

Electrophysiological study and ablation

Electrophysiological study was performed under general anesthesia (propofol). Five multipolar electrode catheters were inserted percutaneously into the right subclavian vein and right and left femoral veins. Three of the catheters were advanced to the right atrial appendage, His bundle region, and coronary sinus. A 7-Fr deflectable catheter with 20 electrodes (Halo catheter; Biosense Webster, Inc) was positioned around the tricuspid annulus (Figure 30.2). A 7.5-Fr catheter with a 3.5-mm-tip electrode (NaviStar ThermoCool; Biosense-Webster, Inc) was used for mapping and ablation. Entrainment pacing (cycle length 15 ms shorter than the tachycardia cycle length) at the lateral right atrium, adjacent to the tricuspid annulus produced manifest fusion and a very long postpacing interval (100 ms longer than the tachycardia cycle length), indicating that the reentrant circuit is not located close to the tricuspid annulus. Limited

Electroanatomical Mapping, 1st edition. Edited by
A. Al-Ahmad, D. Callans, H. Hsia and A. Natale.
© 2008 Blackwell Publishing, ISBN: 9781405157025.

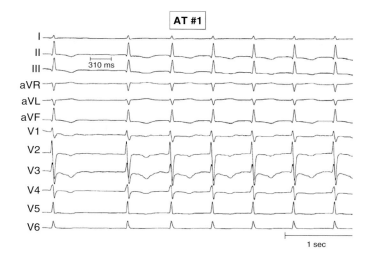

Figure 30.1 The 12-lead electrocardiogram during atrial tachycardia (AT #1) showing very low-voltage P waves with a cycle length of 310 ms.

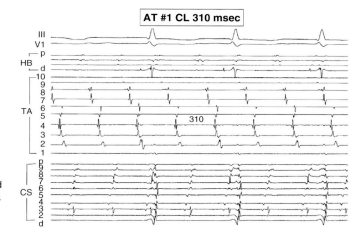

Figure 30.2 Intracardiac electrograms during AT #1 (cycle length 310 ms). Tracings from the top are ECG lead III and V1 and bipolar electrograms from the His bundle region (HB), around the tricuspid annulus (TA) and CS.

electroanatomical mapping (CARTO™) of the right atrium during tachycardia demonstrated earliest right atrial activation at the coronary sinus (CS) ostium, suggesting activation from the left atrium to the right atrium. After trans-septal puncture (8.5-Fr sheath), electroanatomical mapping of the left atrium and each of the four PVs was performed.

An electroanatomical map of the left atrium during AT #1 identified a small macroreentrant circuit around the left inferior pulmonary vein (LIPV) (Figures 30.3 and 30.4). The carina between the left superior PV and the left inferior PV formed the isolated arrhythmogenic channel. PV potentials were recorded in all four PVs and there was no complete conduction block across the mitral isthmus or

between the left and right circumferential PV ablation lines. Linear radiofrequency (RF) ablation between the left inferior PV and the mitral annulus (mitral isthmus ablation line) converted the initial AT to a second macroreentrant left AT (AT #2, cycle length of 370 ms). An electroanatomical map of the left atrium and PVs during AT #2 identified a reentrant circuit with activation propagating around the left superior pulmonary vein (LSPV) and through the carina (Figure 30.5). A single RF application on the carina between the LSPV and LIPV (arrhythmogenic channel) eliminated AT #2 (Figure 30.6). In order to prevent another macroreentrant circuit around the right PVs, seven additional RF applications were delivered along the roof between the RSPV and LSPV (Limited electroanatomical). After ablation, programmed atrial stimulation failed to induce either atrial tachycardia (AT) or atrial fibrillation (AF). During a 3-year follow-up period, the patient has been free of symptomatic episodes of AT or AF without receiving antiarrhythmic medications.

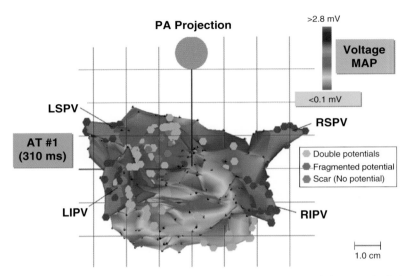

Figure 30.3   Voltage map (posterior-anterior, PA projection) during incessant AT (AT #1) shows markedly low voltage (red, <0.1 mV) with double atrial potentials (pink tags) and fractionated atrial potentials (olive tags) in the posterior left atrium between the right and the left PVs and within the PVs. PV potentials were recorded in all four PVs, indicating incomplete PV isolation.

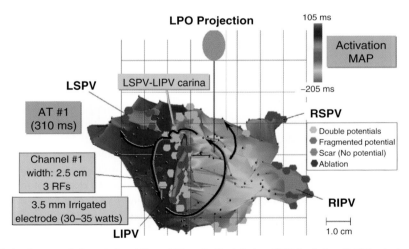

Figure 30.4   Activation map (left posterior oblique, LPO projection) during AT #1 (cycle length 310 ms), demonstrating a small reentrant circuit propagating through the carina between the left superior (LS) PV and left inferior (LI) PV and around the LIPV. RF ablation between the line of conduction block at the anterior margin of the LIPV (a line of pink tags) and the mitral annulus (width 2.5 cm, greatest bipolar voltage 1.48 mV) using three RF applications with a saline irrigated electrode (30–35 W) lengthened the tachycardia cycle length to 370 ms and changed the local atrial activation sequence (AT #2).

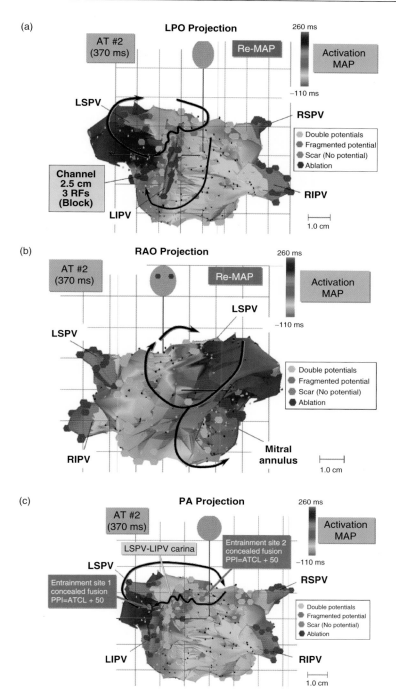

Figure 30.5 Activation map during AT #2 (cycle length 370 ms) in the LPO projection (panel a) and in the right anterior oblique (RAO) projection (panel b), showing continuing activation through the carina between the LSPV and LIPV and around the LSPV. Entrainment pacing (pacing cycle length 355 ms) on both sides of the carina (Entrain Site 1 and Entrain Site 2, panel c) produced the same atrial activation sequence as the tachycardia (concealed fusion). The postpacing interval was the same at both sites (50 ms longer than the tachycardia cycle length), indicating both sites were within (or equally close to) the reentrant circuit, confirming conduction across the carina as the arrhythmogenic channel. The 50 ms delay in the postpacing interval probably resulted from conduction delay within the reentrant circuit produced by entrainment pacing.

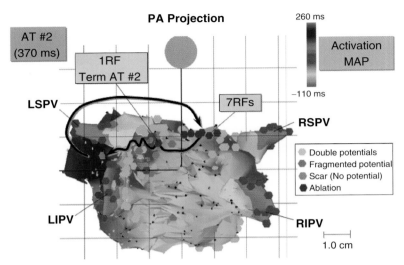

Figure 30.6   A single RF application on the carina between the LSPV and LIPV terminated AT #2. One additional RF application was delivered within the carina, producing complete conduction block between the LSPV and LIPV. Another linear lesion (seven RF applications) was created along the roof between the RSPV and the LSPV to prevent macroreentry around the right PVs.

CHAPTER 31

Macroreentry left atrial tachycardia

Linda Huffer, MD *& William Stevenson,* MD

Clinical vignette

The patient is a male in his sixth decade who had mitral valve repair and surgical atrial MAZE procedure done 3 years ago. Approximately 1 year after surgery, he experienced symptomatic atrial flutter refractory to medical therapy including amiodarone. Electrophysiologic study at that time identified three macroreentrant atrial flutter circuits. One circuit was found to involve the area around the left pulmonary veins where it was interrupted with a line of lesions between the left inferior pulmonary vein and the mitral annulus. A second left atrial flutter circuit revolving around the right pulmonary veins was induced and interrupted with lesions extending from the right veins to the fossa ovalis. Clockwise cavotricuspid isthmus-dependent flutter was also induced and terminated with an ablation line from the tricuspid valve annulus to the inferior vena cava and bidirectional block was confirmed. This procedure was complicated by a left frontal lobe embolus with right arm and leg weakness that subsequently resolved without residual deficit.

He remained in sinus rhythm for only 2 weeks. A cardioversion was performed, which restored sinus rhythm that persisted for almost a year. Atrial arrhythmias subsequently recurred with rapid ventricular response associated with dyspnea and near syncope despite medical therapy. He was then referred for a second catheter ablation procedure which is shown in Figures 31.1–31.10.

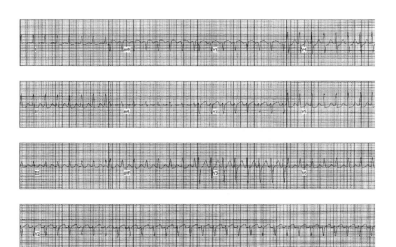

Figure 31.1 Atrial tachycardia/atypical atrial flutter – 12-lead electrocardiogram. The "flutter" waves are obscured by the T wave although suggestive of atypical atrial flutter. Given the clinical history of a prior atrial fibrillation ablation, left atrial macroreentry flutter is the most likely etiology.

Electroanatomical Mapping, 1st edition. Edited by A. Al-Ahmad, D. Callans, H. Hsia and A. Natale. © 2008 Blackwell Publishing, ISBN: 9781405157025.

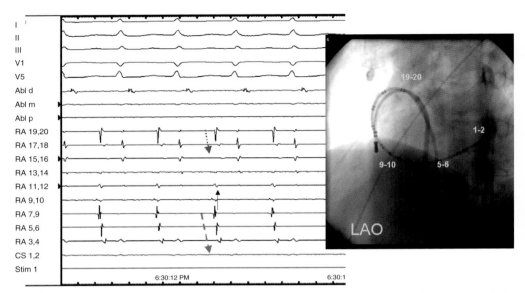

Figure 31.2 Atrial tachycardia/atrial flutter, intracardiac electrograms from the top are surface electrograms lead I, II, III, v1, and v5, bipolar intracardiac electrograms recorded from the ablation catheter (distal, mid, and proximal), and from a 20-pole catheter positioned as shown in the fluoroscopic image (from another patient for illustration purposes). The most proximal electrodes (19–20) are at the high lateral right atrium; the distal electrodes from 5–6 to 1–2 are in the coronary sinus. Many of the atrial signals are low amplitude and the ventricular electrogram is prominent on electrodes 17–18 and 19–20, indicating that the catheter is close to the tricuspid annulus. The lateral wall of the right atrium is activated high to low (blue arrow) and the coronary sinus is activated in a proximal to distal direction (from 5–6 toward 3–4). This suggests common counterclockwise flutter, but the RA subeustachean isthmus is activated in a septal to lateral direction (5–6 is slightly before 9–10), which is not consistent with counterclockwise flutter, but is consistent with isthmus block.

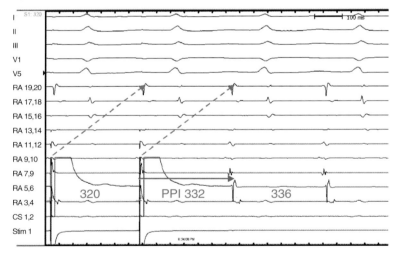

Figure 31.3 Entrainment from the proximal coronary sinus. Tracings are as in Figure 31.2 without the ablation catheter shown. The last two stimuli of a pacing train at a cycle length of 320 ms are shown followed by continuation of the atrial tachycardia at 336 ms. Stimuli delivered from the proximal coronary sinus (RA 5,6) entrain the atrial tachycardia as indicated by acceleration of the atrial electrograms to the pacing rate during stimulation. The postpacing interval (PPI, blue arrow) measured from the last stimulus to the next atrial electrogram on the pacing channel (332 ms) is approximately the tachycardia cycle length, consistent with a reentry circuit site. Note the very long conduction time from the pacing site to the high lateral right atrium (red arrows) consistent with block in the RA subeustachean isthmus. All measurements are in ms.

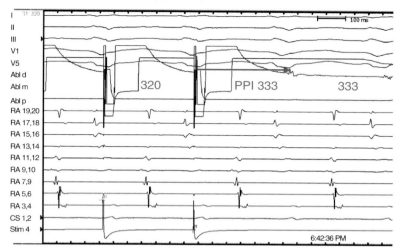

Figure 31.4   Entrainment from the left atrial roof, site 1. Tracings are as in Figure 31.2. The last two stimuli of a pacing train at a cycle length of 320 ms are shown followed by continuation of the atrial tachycardia at a cycle length of 333 ms. Pacing entrains the atrial tachycardia as indicated by acceleration of the atrial electrograms to the pacing rate during stimulation. The PPI (blue arrow) measured from the last stimulus to the next atrial electrogram at the pacing site is equal to the tachycardia cycle length, consistent with a reentry circuit site. Note that the RA activation sequence during LA pacing is the same as during tachycardia, consistent with activation of the RA from the LA during tachycardia.

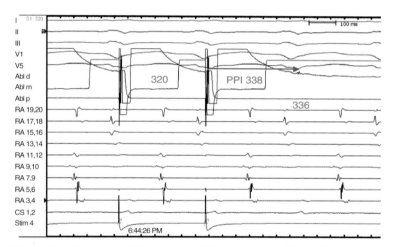

Figure 31.5   Entrainment from the posterior left atrium, site 2. Tracings are as in Figure 31.2. The last two stimuli of a pacing train at a cycle length of 320 ms are shown followed by continuation of the atrial tachycardia at 336 ms. Pacing at the left atrial posterior wall entrains the atrial tachycardia with a PPI measured from the last stimulus to the next atrial electrogram at the pacing site of 338 ms, consistent with a reentry circuit site.

Electrophysiology study and ablation

The patient presented in sinus rhythm with normal conduction intervals. Persistence of bidirectional block across the cavotricuspid isthmus was confirmed with differential atrial pacing. Incremental atrial pacing and double atrial programmed extra-stimuli failed to induce atrial arrhythmias. An iso-proterenol infusion (4 mcg/min) was initiated. Atrial burst pacing at a cycle length of 130 ms then induced atrial fibrillation. Trans-septal puncture was undertaken and an electroanatomic map was obtained using the CARTO™ system and a saline-irrigated mapping and ablation catheter (Thermocool; Biosense Webster, Inc). Atrial fibrillation spontaneously organized to atrial tachycardia (Figure 31.1). Entrainment and activation mapping were then performed.

The tachycardia was stable and regular with a cycle length of 330–340 ms, allowing entrainment to be assessed from selected sites as an electroanatomic map was created. At the proximal coronary sinus, pacing entrained the tachycardia with a post-pacing interval (PPI) similar to that of the tachycardia, indicating that the region was within the reentry circuit. Similarly, entrainment from LA roof (Figure 31.4), posterior wall (Figure 31.5), and in the isthmus between the left inferior pulmonary vein and mitral annulus (Figure 31.6) confirmed that these sites were in the flutter circuit. In contrast, entrainment at the right pulmonary vein produced a longer PPI indicating that the region was remote from the circuit. The activation map

constructed simultaneously (Figure 31.10a and b) was also consistent with macroreentry involving the region between the posterolateral mitral annulus and the left inferior pulmonary veins (mitral isthmus). In addition, a region of electrically unexcitable scar (noncapture with unipolar pacing at 10 mA/2 ms pulse width) was detected at the left inferior pulmonary vein antrum most likely secondary to the patient's previous pulmonary vein isolation. Atrial tachycardia terminated during radiofrequency ablation at the mitral isthmus (Figure 31.7). Additional ablation was applied in a linear fashion until mitral isthmus block was achieved. Bidirectional mitral isthmus block was demonstrated by pacing from the proximal coronary sinus (Figure 31.8) and left atrial appendage (Figure 31.9). No other atrial tachycardias were inducible. The patient had remained free of recurrent arrhythmias as of his last evaluation approximately 2 months after ablation.

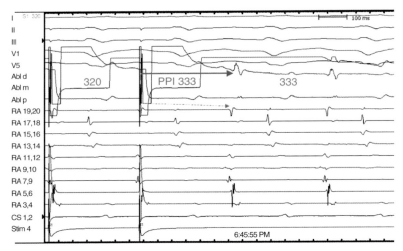

Figure 31.6   Entrainment from the mitral isthmus region, site 3 in Figure 31.10b, between the mitral annulus and left pulmonary veins. Tracings are as in Figure 31.2. The last two stimuli of a pacing train at a cycle length of 320 ms are shown followed by continuation of the atrial tachycardia at 333 ms. Pacing entrains atrial tachycardia as indicated by acceleration of the atrial electrograms to the pacing rate during stimulation. The PPI measured from the last stimulus to the next atrial electrogram at the pacing site (333 ms) is equal to the tachycardia cycle length, consistent with a reentry circuit site. Note the long conduction time from the mitral isthmus to the lateral right atrium consistent with prior surgical and catheter ablation (red arrow).

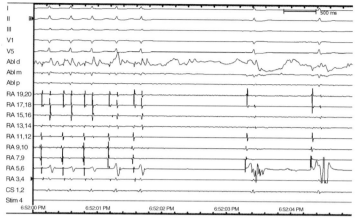

Figure 31.7 Termination of atrial tachycardia during RF ablation, atrial tachycardia terminated during the third radiofrequency ablation lesion at the mitral isthmus. Tachycardia termination was followed by sinus rhythm (last beat depicted). Termination was preceded by cycle length slowing of the two beats prior to termination.

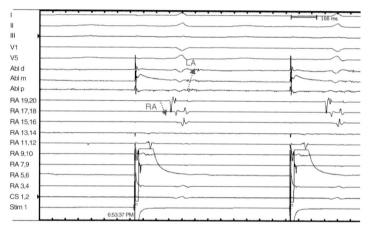

Figure 31.8 Mitral isthmus block assessed by pacing from the proximal coronary sinus. The ablation catheter is positioned above the mitral isthmus line with the distal electrodes closer to the line than the proximal electrodes. Pacing from the proximal coronary sinus demonstrates proximal to distal atrial activation in the ablation catheter consistent with activation approaching the ablation line from above it, consistent with the presence of counterclockwise mitral isthmus block. Also note the right atrial activation sequence, with high to low lateral RA activation consistent with block in the subeustachean isthmus.

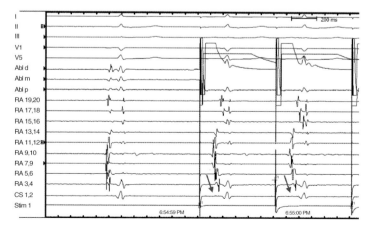

Figure 31.9 Mitral isthmus block evaluated by pacing from the left atrial appendage. The ablation catheter is in the left atrial appendage, above the mitral isthmus block line. During pacing from the left atrial appendage the coronary sinus is activated from proximal to distal (blue arrow) consistent with the presence of clockwise mitral isthmus block.

(a)

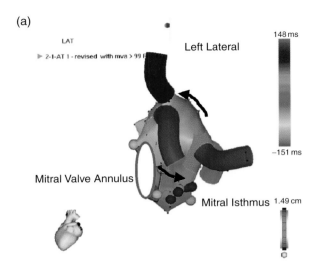

LAT

▶ 2-1-AT 1 - revised with mva > 99 P

Left Lateral

148 ms

−151 ms

Mitral Valve Annulus

Mitral Isthmus 1.49 cm

(b)

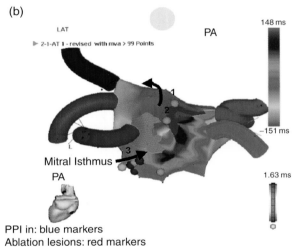

LAT

▶ 2-1-AT 1 - revised with mva > 99 Points

PA

148 ms

−151 ms

Mitral Isthmus

PA

1.63 ms

PPI in: blue markers
Ablation lesions: red markers

Figure 31.10 Atrial tachycardia activation map: left lateral view (a) and PA view (b). Activation proceeds from red, to yellow, to green, to blue, to purple as the wave front proceeds around the left pulmonary veins and up the posterior wall of the left atrium. Note that the activation times color-coded from +148 to −151 ms sum to 299 ms, approximately 88% of the atrial tachycardia cycle length. The earliest and latest sites depicted in red and purple, respectively, meet at the left atrial posterior wall (head meets tail). An area of electrically unexcitable scar (noncapture with unipolar pacing at 10 mA/2 ms pulse width) is shown as the gray region at the antrum of the left inferior pulmonary vein likely due to prior pulmonary vein isolation. Sites where entrainment mapping produced a PPI indicating that the site was in the circuit are indicated with blue circles. Ablation lesion sites are dark red circles.

CHAPTER 32

Focal atrial tachycardia in a patient with a Fontan

John Triedman, MD

Clinical vignette

The patient is a 34-year-old man with atrial tachy-cardia and a history of complex heterotaxy with asplenia. His anatomical malformations include bilateral superior vena cavae, a left-sided inferior vena cava, D-malposition of the great arteries, anomalous pulmonary venous connection to the coronary sinus, and complete AV canal. He has undergone Waterston shunt in the past, and cur-rently has a right-sided bidirectional Glenn anasto-mosis with a left-sided, lateral tunnel Fontan (Figure 32.1). He has had device closure of his Fontan fenestration (1991), and has had multiple coil embolizations of aortopulmonary collaterals. ECG at baseline shows an atrial rhythm of indeter-minate P-wave morphology without pre-excitation (Figure 32.2), but multiple recent tracings have shown an atrial tachycardia with cycle length 300–330 ms, and both 1:1 and 2:1 conduction. The epi-sodes requiring hospital visit and cardioversion had been occurring with increasing frequency prior to ablation, despite therapy with beta-blockade.

Electrophysiology study and ablation

During electrophysiological study, atrial tachycar-dia of cycle length 305 ms was easily induced and terminated with atrial stimulation (Figure 32.3). The AV conduction varied, with conduction seen at 1:1, 2:1, and 4:3. During 1:1 conduction, some

hemodynamic compromise was observed with hypotension. Diltiazem was administered for rate control, and as the ventricular rate decreased, hemodynamics normalized. Mapping of tachycar-dia substrate was performed utilizing the CARTO™ system. Mapping was initially performed exclu-sively within the Fontan baffle (systemic venous atrium). It quickly became clear that only a small portion of the tachycardia cycle length could be mapped from the baffle. A "transeptal" (trans-atrial baffle) puncture was performed to allow access to the left atrium for mapping (Figure 32.4). A trans-baffle puncture was performed using fluo-roscopic guidance, and directed to the pulmonary venous atrium as identified by previous levophase

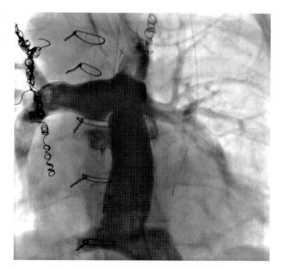

Figure 32.1 AP angiogram of left-sided Fontan baffle, highlighting right PA and including extensive prior embolization of internal mammary arteries for the therapy of pulmonary collaterals.

Electroanatomical Mapping, 1st edition. Edited by A. Al-Ahmad, D. Callans, H. Hsia and A. Natale. © 2008 Blackwell Publishing, ISBN: 9781405157025.

angiography. Although puncture was difficult secondary to extensive calcification of the baffle, ultimately it was performed successfully and without complication by probing several candidate puncture sites to identify a vulnerable point on the baffle. A long sheath was then passed through the puncture site, allowing for mapping within the pulmonary venous atrium. Of note, a postcatheterization echo in this case revealed no residual right-to-left shunt after catheterization (Figure 32.5); in other cases, small residual shunts are observed after such procedures. The tachycardia was mapped to a focal area in the right lateral posterior region; in normal cardiac anatomy, this would correspond to

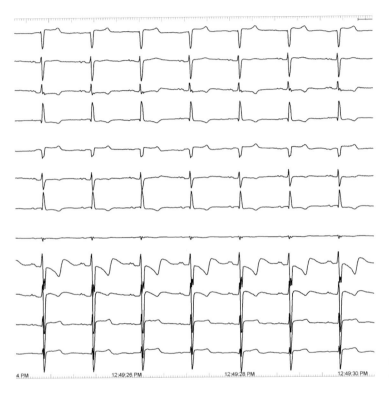

Figure 32.2 "Sinus" rhythm observed at start of case.

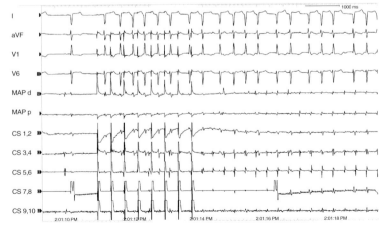

Figure 32.3 Atrial tachycardia induced by atrial extrastimuli.

the region of the normal sinus node (Figure 32.6). The focal origin of the tachycardia, in combination with the tachycardia's response to atrial extrastimuli, suggested a focal atrial reentrant tachycardia. Ablation was performed during tachycardia, with prompt cessation of tachycardia (Figure 32.7). Because of low power input and high temperatures noted on the initial lesion, the ablation catheter was changed to an irrigated catheter, and 11 additional

lesions were placed. Following these lesions, tachycardia could not be induced, with and without isuprel infusion. Although not common, focal atrial tachycardias are well described in the population of patients with congenital heart disease. These arrhythmias are of uncertain mechanism. However, they most likely represent a microreentrant mechanism, as they display a focal, radial activation pattern and are typically easily and reproducibly initiated and terminated by atrial pacing. This case demonstrates the limited access that may be available for mapping and ablating congenital heart patients due to surgically created intraatrial obstacles such as baffles. In some patients, it may be possible to effect catheter placement via a retrograde

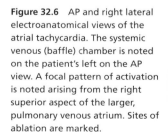

Figure 32.4 Placement of a transeptal sheath across the Fontan baffle to the pulmonary venous "right" atrium. The baffle is pierced just superior and posterior to the occlusive device used previously to close the surgical fenestration. The ablation catheter sits in the site of successful ablation; compared with the mapped site of ablation in Figure 32.6. A decapolar catheter is placed in the baffle for use as an electrogram reference.

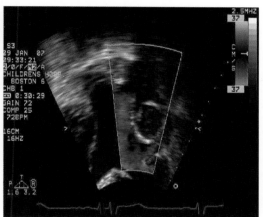

Figure 32.5 Postcatheterization Doppler echocardiogram showing a transverse cut of the oval baffle, and absence of any residual shunting at the site of the transeptal puncture.

Figure 32.6 AP and right lateral electroanatomical views of the atrial tachycardia. The systemic venous (baffle) chamber is noted on the patient's left on the AP view. A focal pattern of activation is noted arising from the right superior aspect of the larger, pulmonary venous atrium. Sites of ablation are marked.

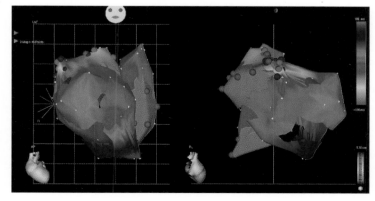

approach, but it is important to recognize that the geometry of semilunar and AV valves may preclude this, or render it so awkward as to be useless. Use of transeptal techniques to provide access across surgical baffles has been reported, and this technique is used frequently in our laboratory. A biplane levophase angiogram is used to plan and guide needle placement, and a systematic exploration of the baffle often reveals a "weak spot," which can be traversed without excessive force.

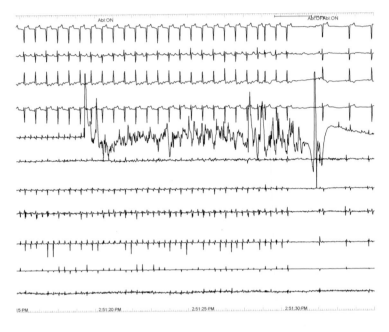

Figure 32.7 Rapid termination of tachycardia at the onset of the first radiofrequency application.

CHAPTER 33

Macroreentrant atrial tachycardia in patient with a history of tetralogy of Fallot

John Triedman, MD

Clinical vignette

The patient is a 25-year-old young woman with a history of tetralogy of Fallot, for which she initially underwent Waterston shunt, followed by a Blalock-Taussig shunt, and finally a complete trans-annular patch repair at the age of 3. She has a history of recurrent atrial tachycardia despite medical therapy. Prior cardioversion had resulted in prolonged asystole followed by profound bradycardia, necessitating resuscitation. On tachycardia recurrence, she was referred for electrophysiological study and ablation.

Her most recent cardiac MRI, in January 2005, demonstrated biventricular dysfunction with LV ejection fraction of 43%, and only mild right atrial dilation. Pulmonary regurgitant fraction was 10%. An echocardiogram performed on the day of electrophysiological study demonstrated low-normal LV function (LV ejection fraction of 54%), mildly depressed RV function, and an estimated RV pressure ~40 mmHg. Electrocardiogram on admission showed an atrial tachycardia with cycle length approximately 275 ms and variable AV conduction (Figure 33.1).

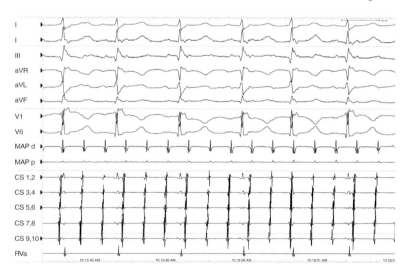

Figure 33.1 Atrial tachycardia at the onset of the study. Although the electrocardiogram is not suggestive of typical atrial flutter, the P-wave axis and proximal-to-distal electrogram progression in the coronary sinus wire suggest a right atrial origin of the tachycardia.

Electroanatomical Mapping, 1st edition. Edited by
A. Al-Ahmad, D. Callans, H. Hsia and A. Natale.
© 2008 Blackwell Publishing, ISBN: 9781405157025.

Electrophysiology study and ablation

As is typically the practice in our laboratory, a right atrial angiography was performed to delineate right atrial anatomy; the atrium was moderately dilated, but otherwise appeared grossly normal (Figure 33.2). Electroanatomical mapping was commenced while in tachycardia. During mapping, catheter manipulation within the right atrium resulted in termination of tachycardia. A prolonged sinus pause (> 3 s) was seen, with resumption of slow sinus rhythm. In order to continue mapping, tachycardia was restarted with rapid atrial pacing; confirmation that the original tachycardia has been re-induced is made by cycle length and P-wave morphology. Mapping revealed a macroreentrant circuit that utilized the lateral right atrial wall and revolved horizontally around the right atrium (Figure 33.3). The borders of this protected corridor are not clearly determined, but the superior line of absent electrograms (gray tags and tissue = "scar") or double potentials (pale blue tags) suggest the involvement of an atriotomy, bypass cannulation sites, and/or the crista terminalis. Although mapping of bipolar electrode voltage sometimes reveals an anatomical signature, in this patient, low-amplitude electrograms were diffuse and did not contribute

to prediction or understanding of the circuit (Figure 33.4). Radiofrequency (RF) ablation was initiated in this region with an irrigated RF ablation catheter. Termination of tachycardia occurred during the first RF lesion, preceded by gradual cycle

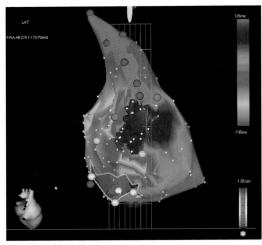

Figure 33.3 Right lateral (and slightly posterior) view of the lateral free wall corridor supporting the tachycardia present in this patient. Activation proceeds horizontally around the atrium, moving medial to lateral on the anterior surface and lateral to medial on the posterior.

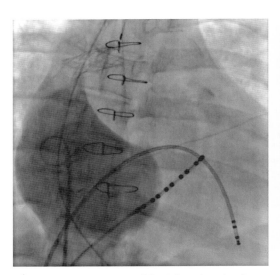

Figure 33.2 AP angiogram of the right atrium showing mild enlargement, and stenting of the right proximal PA for relieve of postoperative stenosis.

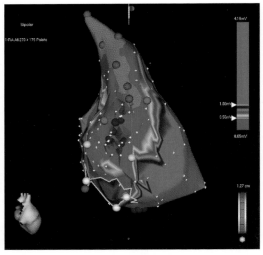

Figure 33.4 Bipolar voltage map in the same view, showing that most of the atrial endocardial surface registers electrograms below a commonly used voltage threshold for denoting "scar tissue" (0.50 mV).

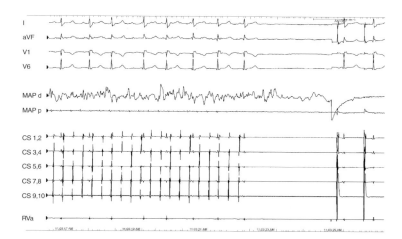

Figure 33.5 Termination of the clinical atrial tachycardia with ablation is often preceded by cycle length prolongation.

length prolongation of ~30 ms (Figure 33.5). Marked sinus node dysfunction with intermittent asystolic pauses was again seen following termination of tachycardia, and the remainder of the case would be performed while the patient was atrially paced. Additional lesions were placed to create a line of block along the lateral right atrium. Owing to some catheter instability, a directional sheath (Daig SAFL curve) was utilized to help guide and control the catheter along the lateral right atrial wall. Although mapping did not reveal a circuit involving the cavotricuspid isthmus, an empiric isthmus block was performed, using nine RF applications. On remapping during atrial pacing from the proximal coronary sinus, isthmus block was incomplete, with breakthrough activation at the caval end of the ablation line (Figure 33.6). After additional lesions were applied, pacing both at the ostium of the coronary sinus and in the low lateral right atrium between the isthmus and lateral free wall ablation lines revealed conduction block at both sites (Figure 33.7). Tachycardia could not be re-induced with atrial pacing or atrial extrastimuli. A transvenous dual chamber pacemaker was subsequently implanted at a separate procedure. In patients with biventricular forms of congenital heart disease, the most common anatomical substrate for atrial tachycardia is the isthmus between the inferior vena cava and the right-sided AV valve, as is the case in normal cardiac anatomy. However, atypical circuits are frequently encountered, and abnormalities of atrial mass and anatomy often

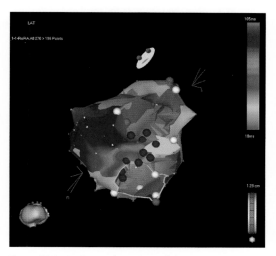

Figure 33.6 Pacing at the ostium of the coronary sinus after attempted creation of cavotricuspid isthmus block, view in left anterior oblique (LAO) and inferior projection, shows a green area of breakthrough at the caval end of the line, and latest activation distant from the edge of the ablation line.

result in activation patterns that make diagnosis of typical atrial flutter difficult. In this patient, an empiric isthmus block is necessary because of the high likelihood that she will have flutter anchored to that feature in the future. The standard procedural endpoint for ablation of atrial flutter is demonstration of isthmus block. This is also desirable to ascertain in atypical atrial tachycardia circuits such as this one. In many cases, however, identification of a suitable pacing site to investigate this is difficult. Ideally, pacing should be performed as close to the ablated site as possible, and conduction on the opposite side of the line of lesions should show no signs of early breakthrough at all.

This study demonstrates the anatomical utility of careful mapping "downstream" from the line of ablation; mapping of early breakthrough directed additional lesions to be performed near the cavoatrial junction.

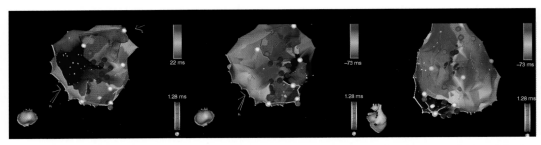

Figure 33.7   After completion of the caval end of the line, latest activation is seen at the "downstream" edge of the line during pacing at the coronary sinus as well as the low lateral right atrium. In addition, the right frame shows similar evidence of block at the free wall ablation line.

CHAPTER 34

Double loop macroreentrant atrial tachycardia in a patient with tetralogy of Fallot

John Triedman, MD

Clinical vignette

The patient is a 26-year-old man with history of Trisomy 21 and tetralogy of Fallot. He initially underwent complete repair of his tetralogy using a trans-annular patch, and was subsequently re-operated for placement of a valved right ventricle to pulmonary artery conduit to address right ventricular failure associated with severe pulmonary insufficiency. Echocardiogram at the time of referral revealed moderate right ventricular outflow tract obstruction, mild pulmonary regurgitation, and moderate tricuspid regurgitation. The right ventricle was dilated, with qualitatively mild dysfunction and a pressure estimated by Doppler interrogation to be 78 mmHg above right atrial. Left ventricular function was qualitatively normal. In addition to his hemodynamic residua, he has undergone DDD-pacemaker implantation for sinus node dysfunction and second-degree AV block. Over the 3 years prior to this study, he developed recurrent atrial tachycardia, which has required DC cardioversion on multiple occasions.

Electrophysiology study and ablation

The baseline electrocardiogram demonstrated a dual-chamber-paced rhythm. Initial angiography demonstrated total occlusion of the inferior vena cava, necessitating a catheter approach based on subclavian and internal jugular venous access (Figure 34.1). Hemodynamic evaluation was performed, and there was no residual intracardiac shunting, with a mean right atrial pressure of 12 mmHg. Pulmonary capillary wedge pressure was 10. The patient's pacemaker was changed from DDD-pacing to VVI (backup) pacing, revealing slow underlying sinus rhythm (Figure 34.2). The study was performed with a 6-Fr decapolar deflectable catheter in the right atrium as a reference catheter, and a 7-Fr CARTO™ catheter as a mapping/ablation catheter. An esophageal lead was passed for additional monitoring of atrial activation.

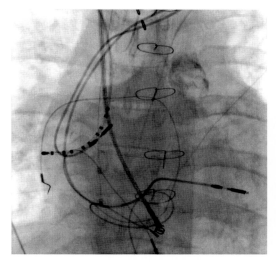

Figure 34.1 Positions of catheters placed in subclavian and internal jugular positions, as well as active transvenous and abandoned epicardial pacing leads. Note the position of a bipolar trans-esophageal catheter to the right of the patient's spine at the level of the low left atrium.

Electroanatomical Mapping, 1st edition. Edited by A. Al-Ahmad, D. Callans, H. Hsia and A. Natale. © 2008 Blackwell Publishing, ISBN: 9781405157025.

Electroanatomical mapping was first performed in sinus rhythm. An atrial tachycardia was then induced using atrial extrastimuli, with a cycle length of 225 ms and variable, slow AV conduction (Figure 34.3). Mapping during tachycardia revealed a circuit that appeared to form a double-loop or "figure-of-eight" pattern utilizing both the cavotricuspid isthmus and a narrow corridor of tissue at the lateral border of the right atrium and the inferior vena cava (Figure 34.4). A voltage map of the lateral right atrium demonstrates the presumed area of scarring and low voltage that anchors the lateral loop; this may be related to surgical scarring,

fibrosis and hypertrophy, and/or poor transverse electrical conduction across the crista terminalis (Figure 34.5). Radiofrequency (RF) applications were initially created at the cavotricuspid isthmus. During the fourth application, acceleration of the tachycardia with alteration of the P-wave morphology was seen (Figure 34.6). This was subsequently followed by sudden termination during further ablation, and tachycardia was not inducible for the remainder of the case (Figure 34.7).

A total of 27 RF lesions were created within the isthmus and in the more posterior and lateral region, creating two distinct lines of ablation.

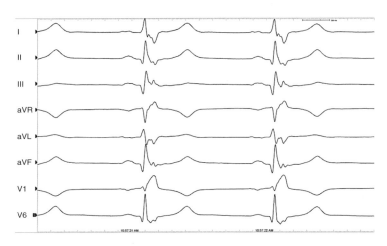

Figure 34.2 Underlying sinus rhythm at the start of the case.

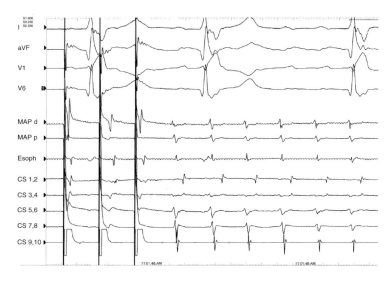

Figure 34.3 Induction of clinical tachycardia.

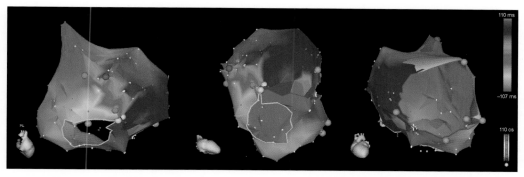

Figure 34.4 Double-loop tachycardia. Left panel: right lateral view, showing lateral wall loop with lower turnaround at the right atrial inferior vena caval margin. Blue tags represent double-potential recordings, gray indicates scar, and pink, long, fractionated potentials. Middle panel: inferior view, showing tachycardia activation progressing down the anterolateral margin of the tricuspid annulus and bifurcating around the lateral wall (left) and the cavotricuspid isthmus (right). Right panel: left oblique view presenting the peri-annular component of the tachycardia, with the tricuspid annulus en face.

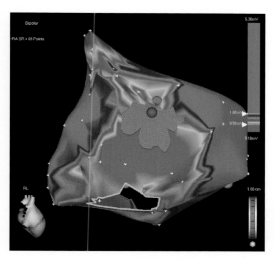

Figure 34.5 Voltage map of the lateral right atrium, showing diffuse area of low voltage (red) and absent voltage (gray) on the lateral wall.

At first remapping, activation sequences seen during lateral atrial pacing suggested that a residual corridor of conduction existed in the cavotricuspid isthmus (Figure 34.8). The suspect area was subjected to further ablation at the tricuspid annulus, and at the conclusion of the case, remapping convincingly demonstrated conduction block across both lines (Figure 34.9). Knowledge of prior surgical and catheter-based interventions in patients with congenital heart disease is important

for procedure planning even in patients who are essentially "fixed" anatomically (i.e., biventricular repair without residual septal defects). In this patient, prior interventions had resulted in interruption of standard femoral venous access, and a modified catheter approach (access from above, with the use of an ancillary esophageal electrode for atrial synchronization) was necessary. Double-loop or "figure-of-eight" tachycardias have been frequently described. These tachycardias usually involve the right-sided AV annulus and an area of scarring on the lateral right atrium to define the two loops, with the common isthmus composed of the corridor of atrial myocardium between the two obstacles. Although ablation at this common isthmus (in this case, lateral to the tricuspid annulus) might theoretically seem to be the most efficient way of addressing both circuits, practically it may be easier to ablate at two targets that are more easily ablated. It is not uncommon to see that ablation in congenital heart disease results in abrupt prolongation of tachycardia cycle length without termination; in these cases, remapping often reveals the subsidiary loop, which must then be interrupted to complete the procedure. In this patient, an abrupt decrease in tachycardia cycle length was noted with change in the P-wave morphology during ablation – this is an atypical response and not explained by the mechanisms postulated above, nor by other data available in this

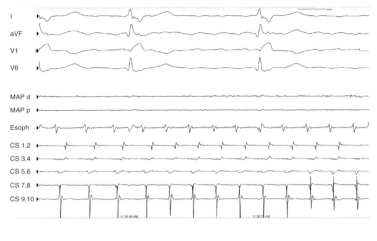

Figure 34.6   Acceleration of atrial tachycardia cycle length during ablation of the cavotricuspid isthmus, with apparent change in P-wave morphology.

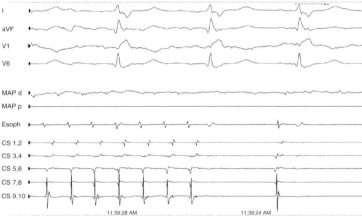

Figure 34.7   Termination of faster tachycardia during the next subsequent ablation at the isthmus. Spontaneous termination of tachycardia unrelated to RF application cannot be ruled out.

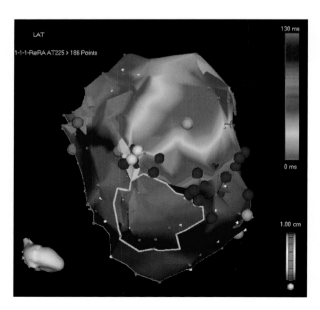

Figure 34.8   Pace-mapping from low lateral right atrium after ablation at both corridors. Note that while the lateral corridor is blocked, the isthmus to the right shows earlier activation (pale blue) than the posterior atrium (deep blue to purple), which can only arise if there is conduction across the ablated area.

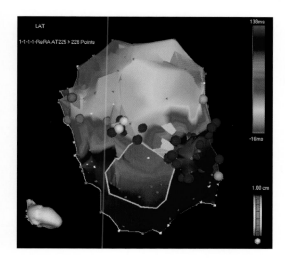

Figure 34.9 Mapping after additional lesions now shows latest activation just opposite the ablation line at the isthmus. Differences in color scale compared to last figure reflect (a) different pacing location, (b) less attention paid to mapping lateral isthmus block, and (c) autoscale effects of color bar by electroanatomical mapping system.

case. Although scouting for complete block of the cavotricuspid isthmus by pace-mapping is a well-established technique for ablation of atrial flutter, it is often difficult to clearly ascertain block in patients with congenital heart disease. In this study, the signs of an "open" isthmus on electro-anatomical remap are demonstrated, and an example of the data obtained during remapping of a more atypically located conduction corridor is presented.

CHAPTER 35

Atrial flutter in a patient post-Fontan

John Triedman, MD

Clinical vignette

The patient is a 19-year-old young woman with a history of double-inlet left ventricle, straddling tricuspid valve, and large perimembranous VSD and normally related great arteries. She underwent a Fontan procedure in 1990 in London. That procedure involved surgical creation of an atriopulmonary anastomosis, and pericardial patch septation of the right atrium, closing the small tricuspid valve from all venous flow other than those that drained from the coronary sinus into a small chamber above the tricuspid valve. She subsequently developed atrial tachycardia, and an attempt at catheter ablation was made in London in 2005 but was unsuccessful. Tachycardia has persisted despite therapy with amiodarone. She presented for hemodynamic and electrophysiological studies and planned ablation. Hemodynamic evaluation was intended to determine indications and clinical suitability for possible revision of her circulation to a variation of the total cavopulmonary Fontan, with simultaneous creation of an atrial maze if necessary. Echocardiogram performed prior to the procedure revealed moderate right atrial dilation, and unobstructed right superior vena cava. The small tricuspid valve was regurgitant. A cardiac MRI was also performed, revealing mild right atrial dilation with patent Fontan pathway, a grossly dilated coronary sinus, and a small, supratricuspid chamber

into which the coronary sinus appeared to drain (Figure 35.1).

Electrophysiology study and ablation

Baseline electrocardiogram demonstrated atrial tachycardia with atrial cycle length 280 ms and variable AV conduction resulting in a ventricular rate of 110 bpm (Figure 35.2). Hemodynamic evaluation showed aortic and left ventricular saturation to be 93% and mixed venous saturation 61%, with no step-up in saturation to suggest left-to-right shunting. Cardiac index was 2 L/min/m^2. The mean pressure throughout the Fontan circuit (right atrium and bilateral pulmonary arteries) was 15–16 mmHg. The pulmonary capillary wedge pressure and left ventricular end diastolic pressure were 11–12 mmHg, yielding a trans-pulmonary gradient of 4 mmHg, and pulmonary vascular resistance of 2 Woods units. Anatomical data from cardiac MRI were segmented into the following chambers: right atrium (including atriopulmonary anastomosis and proximal pulmonary arteries), left atrium, coronary sinus, ventricle, and aorta (Figure 35.3). These data were imported and incorporated into the subsequent electroanatomical mapping by coregistration of the segmented and mapped volumes by identification of landmark points for alignment of the images at the proximal right and left pulmonary arteries and the inferoseptal right atrium. Electroanatomical mapping of the right atrium strongly suggested that this was counterclockwise, cavotricuspid isthmus-dependent flutter, but a significant portion of the

Electroanatomical Mapping, 1st edition. Edited by A. Al-Ahmad, D. Callans, H. Hsia and A. Natale. © 2008 Blackwell Publishing, ISBN: 9781405157025.

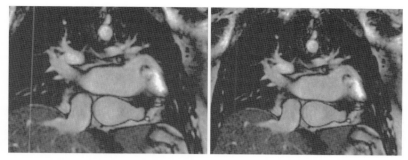

Figure 35.1   Transverse MRI of the atrial structures in this patient. The left frame is approximately 1 cm anterior to the right frame. It shows the moderately dilated right atrium and the ventricular outflow. A small circular chamber is noted adjacent to the inferoseptal aspect of the right atrium; this is a surgically related supratricuspid chamber, draining into the ventricle via a small and indistinctly imaged tricuspid valve. In the right frame, which is posterior to the left, the left atrial chamber is seen superiorly. Beneath this to patients right is the inferior right atrium and confluence of inferior vena cava with hepatic veins; to patient's midline and left is the enormously dilated coronary sinus. This is connected to the supratricuspid chamber by a narrow neck (not imaged).

Figure 35.2   Electrocardiogram of atrial tachycardia at presentation. P waves are prolonged and indistinct, but appear to be separated by an isoelectric interval suggesting the presence of a protected zone of slower conduction.

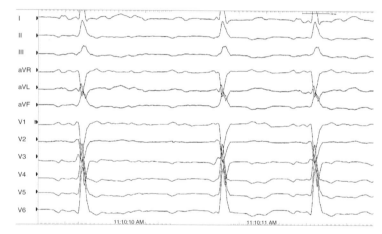

Figure 35.3   AP (left) and PA (right) views of the segmented MRI after integration with the initial electroanatomical map. Coregistration "flags" have been chosen at sites that are well separated in space and reliably and uniquely identifiable in both maps. The right atrium is shown in blue, along with overlay of activation map. The ventricle is purple, left atrium is red, coronary sinus is green, and aorta is pink.

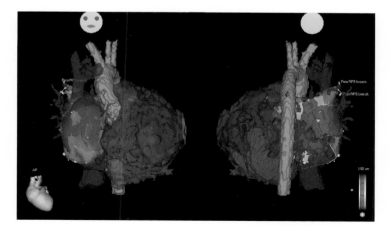

cycle length of the tachycardia was unaccounted for in the map (Figure 35.4). Given the prior MRI data, it appeared that the remainder of the circuit lay on the tricuspid side of the pericardial patch. Performance of postpacing intervals showed that the right atrial side on either side of this patch was clearly "in circuit", with a difference between the postpacing interval and the tachycardia cycle length of ~0 (Figure 35.5). Transeptal puncture was performed to access this small chamber and passage of the dilator and sheath were made possible by dilation of the wire track using a 4-mm cutting balloon. The long sheath (8-Fr) was then passed across the patch (Figure 35.6). Transduction of pressure revealed chamber pressure to be approximately two-third of the systemic level, suggesting significant tricuspid regurgitation and angiography demonstrated that were in fact in the small, distinct chamber just above the tricuspid valve, which had been seen on cardiac MRI. It also became obvious that the coronary sinus was connected to this chamber by a narrow neck, and appeared to decompress via other Thebesian veins. Ablation was initially attempted in this chamber, along the septal patch in the region of the isthmus (Figure 35.7). Because of the small size of the chamber and the tricuspid inlet, it was difficult to maneuver the catheters in such a way that the terminal curve could be utilized effectively to place the tip on the presumptive area of isthmus conduction. Although transient, slight prolongation of atrial

cycle length was observed, the tachycardia persisted despite the following maneuvers: use of irrigated ablation, use of small-diameter/small-radius ablation catheter, use of bidirectional catheter, approach to ablation site from the internal jugular, and

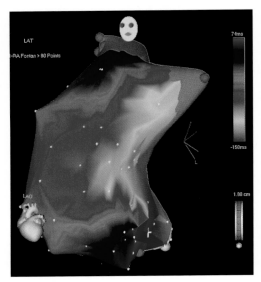

Figure 35.4 Left anterior oblique (LAO) view of the initial map of the right atrium in tachycardia. Note that while there appears to be a counterclockwise loop of activation that utilizes the inferoseptal atrium in the area of the small tricuspid annulus, examination of the time scale on the color bar reveals that only 225 ms of the total cycle length of 280 ms is accounted for, suggesting that a portion of the circuit between purple and red is still undiscovered.

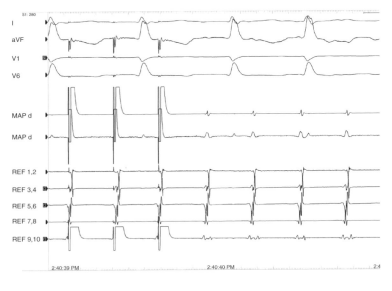

Figure 35.5 A postpacing interval performed just posterior to the isthmus in the right atrium (red area, Figure 35.4), which shows that this area is "in circuit".

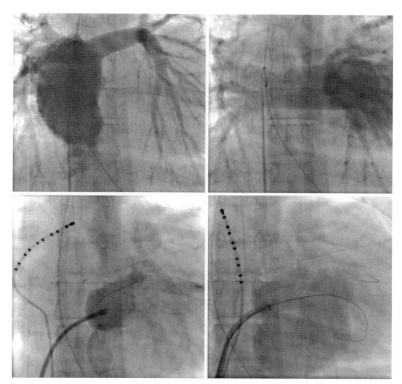

Figure 35.6 Angiographic characterization of atrial chambers, all in AP view. Upper left, right atrium, and Fontan anastomosis. Upper right, left atrium during angiographic levophase. Lower left, supratricuspid chamber via transeptal sheath; note the guide wire traversing tricuspid valve into ventricle to secure position. Lower right, dilated coronary sinus below supratricuspid chamber, note the magnified view.

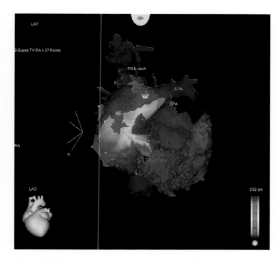

Figure 35.7 Mapping of supratricuspid chamber via transeptal approach shows that the rest of the cycle length of the tachycardia is now accounted for. Also demonstrated is the very small size of this chamber, and its anatomical relation to the coronary sinus (green) and the left atrium (red).

ablation on the right atrial side of the patch. We considered mapping the enlarged coronary sinus. However, the coronary sinus ostium was severely stenosed, and catheter course from the patch through that narrow and acutely angled opening was impossible to achieve. We then set out to create a posterior septal line of block across the isthmus, from the right side of the septal patch. Remapping following these ablations demonstrated apparent change in atrial activation, but it was not possible to terminate the tachycardia. Further attempts at ablation were abandoned at this point, and the atrial tachycardia was easily terminated with rapid atrial pacing. Procedure duration was approximately 7 h. The evolution of electroanatomical mapping, coregistration of anatomical images, response to overdrive pacing, and irrigated ablation were all applied to this patient, and formed what appeared to be a comprehensive picture integrating the patient's unusual anatomy and its relation to the tachycardia circuit. Despite our advanced knowledge in this case, we were unable to terminate what appeared to be an unusual presentation of a common form of tachycardia. Thinking about the specific factors that might have contributed to the failure of this ablation is useful in thinking about what additional innovations might still contribute to expanding the indications for and efficacy of this procedure. Although we had a very clear understanding of this patient's anatomy, the specific, local anatomy of the targeted area was inferred – a currently available technology that may have assisted with this problem would have been the addition of intracardiac ultrasound. Also, manipulation of catheters in small spaces and around tight angles was clearly limiting to the placement of lesions in locations selected by the operator, and it is possible that recently developed technologies using floppy, magnetically guided catheters might have been able to address that specific problem.

CHAPTER 36

Atrial tachycardia in a patient post Mustard procedure

John Triedman, MD

Clinical vignette

The patient is a 46-year-old man with frequent episodes of atrial tachycardia in the setting of transposition of the great arteries' status post Mustard procedure. Poor tricuspid (systemic) valve function prompted surgical tricuspid valvuloplasty with implantation of a Charpentier ring. He also had a prior history of syncope and inducible ventricular tachycardia, and is status post implantation of a dual-chamber implantable cardioverter defibrillator (ICD). Episodes have persisted despite prophylactic medical therapy, and tachycardia is usually resistant to overdrive pacing with pacemaker telemetry, rendering anti-tachycardia pacing (ATP) therapies of limited value and necessitating frequent direct current (DC) cardioversions.

Electrophysiology study and ablation

The patient was initially in atrial-paced rhythm. A pre-ablation angiogram of the neo-right atrium was performed to guide catheter navigation (Figure 36.1). Atrial tachycardia at cycle length 345 ms with 2:1 conduction was easily and repeatedly induced during an atrial stimulation protocol (Figure 36.2). Electroanatomical mapping was performed in atrial tachycardia (Figure 36.3). The catheter used for reference and simple atrial pacing is placed across the inferior limb baffle to the left

Electroanatomical Mapping, 1st edition. Edited by
A. Al-Ahmad, D. Callans, H. Hsia and A. Natale.
© 2008 Blackwell Publishing, ISBN: 9781405157025.

atrial appendage. This position is relatively secure, and if the catheter is dislodged, it can be easily reproduced. Because of the irregularity of the shape of the neo-right atrium, and the tendency of surface-rendering algorithms to smooth acute indentations, separate chambers are created to represent the superior vena caval baffle, the inferior vena cava baffle and mitral inflow, the coronary sinus, and the pulmonary venous atrium. Access to the

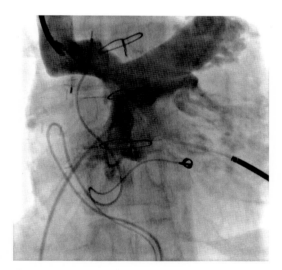

Figure 36.1 AP view of an angiogram of this patient performed to assist in catheter guidance, which shows the typical "pair-of-pants" arrangement typically seen in patients with the Mustard procedure. The SVC-to-mitral baffle limb and the left atrial appendage are well opacified, while the IVC-to-mitral baffle is less well visualized. In addition to trans-venous leads utilized by the patient's current dual-chamber ICD, abandoned epicardial leads are also seen. Finally, a small superior limb baffle leak has previously been closed using a percutaneously placed device.

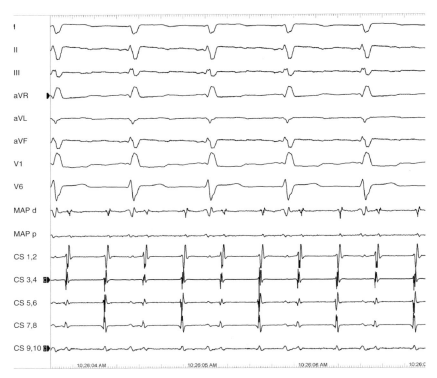

Figure 36.2 Atrial tachycardia induced and mapped in this patient. Note that in many patients with this anatomical arrangement, the coronary sinus is not directly accessible from the neo-right atrium.

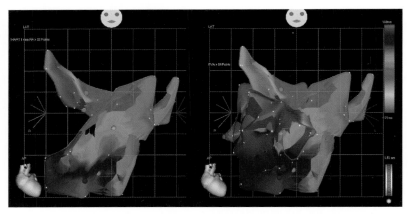

Figure 36.3 AP views of electroanatomical mapping of isthmus-dependent flutter in a patient with a Mustard procedure. In order to define the complex geometry of systemic and pulmonary pathways, it is desirable to use multiple small chambers, avoiding geometrical interpolation and smoothing and preserving anatomical fidelity. In the left panel, the neo-right atrium alone is shown, while the right panel overlies the pulmonary venous atrium and shows the approximate location of the tricuspid valve. Color coding indicates the presence of a clockwise flutter circuit, and ablations made in the isthmus (located principally on the pulmonary venous side of the baffle) terminated the arrhythmia.

pulmonary venous atrium, which connects the pulmonary venous confluence to the tricuspid annulus by wrapping around the "crotch" of the Mustard "pants," was achieved via trans-baffle puncture (Figure 36.4). This patient was noted to have a clockwise atrial flutter around the surgically modified tricuspid annulus, best mapped from within the pulmonary venous atrium. The tachycardia was easily treated with ablation at this site, with slowing of the cycle length prior to termination (Figure 36.5). Creation of conduction block

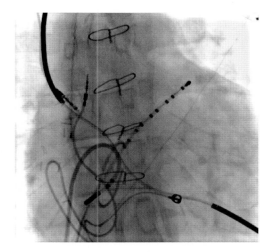

Figure 36.4 An 8-mm-tip radiofrequency mapping and ablation catheter has been placed across the intraatrial baffle using a sheath, with the tip deflected anteriorly and downward to map and ablate on the tricuspid annulus.

along the isthmus (Figure 36.6) and noninducibility of atrial tachycardia were demonstrated. As with tetralogy of Fallot, the biventricular anatomy associated with trans-position of the great arteries makes the right-sided cavotricuspid isthmus a primary substrate for atrial tachycardia in patients who have undergone the Mustard procedure and its relative, the Senning procedure, even though the circuit is largely located on the pulmonary venous side of the surgically created baffle in this and most patients. In general, if an inferior caval vessel is present along with an ipsilateral AV valve, the isthmus created by these structures is likely to be a tachycardia substrate, regardless of whether the valve is tricuspid or mitral, and located on the systemic or pulmonary venous side.

Another important secondary site for tachycardias in these patients is on the lateral atrial free wall, where atriotomies and, often, surgical augmentation of the atrial wall have been performed. Despite the accuracy with which the catheter tip can be tracked using electroanatomical techniques, significant errors in surface reconstruction may be introduced by the parameters used by the device to interpolate between widely scattered points. Practically, this seems to be especially problematic when the operator is trying to define elongated chambers extending off another cardiac chamber. Although the Mustard procedure is an excellent demonstration of this, a more common application is accurate definition and mapping of the proximal pulmonary venous structures.

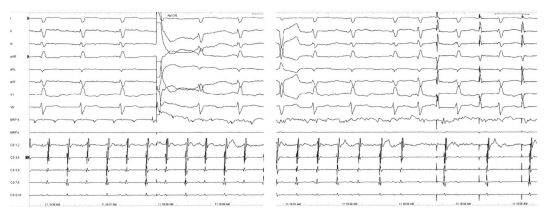

Figure 36.5 Termination of atrial tachycardia with modest prolongation of cycle length (~35 ms) prior to cessation and default to atrial pacing.

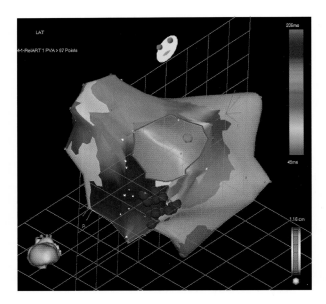

Figure 36.6 Demonstration of postablation conduction block in the pulmonary venous atrium of this patient. The patient is being paced on the atrial septum near the mouth of coronary sinus. Activation swings superior and posteriorly around the heart to activate the lateral isthmus last, indicated by the steady progression to deep blue and purple on the "downstream" side of the ablation line.

CHAPTER 37

Repeat interruption of ongoing atrial fibrillation during RF pulse delivery

Riccardo Cappato, MD

Clinical vignette

A 58-year-old male with recurrent multiple episodes of drug refractory (including amiodarone) idiopathic atrial fibrillation was referred for trans-catheter ablation of the underlying substrate. Atrial fibrillation was initially documented 5 years before referral, became more frequent during the last year with persistent atrial fibrillation refractory to multiple attempts at electrical cardioversion for termination during the last month.

Electrophysiology study and ablation

Catheter ablation was performed using a CARTO™ merge technique for electroanatomical reconstruction of the left atrium and the lasso-assisted catheter technique for guiding electrical disconnection of pulmonary veins. The patient presented at the electrophysiology lab with atrial fibrillation, and multiple attempts at electrical cardioversion failed to restore stable sinus rhythm because of early recurrence of atrial fibrillation (Figure 37.1).

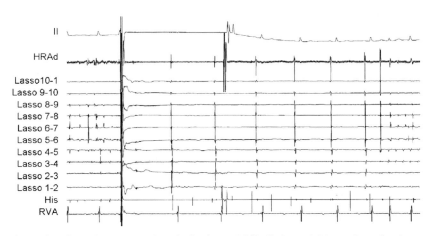

Figure 37.1 Electrical cardioversion restores sinus rhythm but atrial fibrillation re-initiates after a few beats.

Electroanatomical Mapping, 1st edition. Edited by
A. Al-Ahmad, D. Callans, H. Hsia and A. Natale.
© 2008 Blackwell Publishing, ISBN: 9781405157025.

Because of inability to maintain sinus rhythm, isolation of pulmonary veins was initially attempted during atrial fibrillation. Following isolation of the inferior lateral pulmonary vein, RF pulse delivery at the crista between the anterior rim of the superior lateral pulmonary vein and the posterior rim of the entrance of the left appendage (Figure 37.2) resulted in multiple terminations of ongoing atrial fibrillation (Figure 37.3) until sinus rhythm was steadily maintained (Figure 37.4). Sinus rhythm remained throughout the remaining procedure until isolation of all pulmonary veins was obtained.

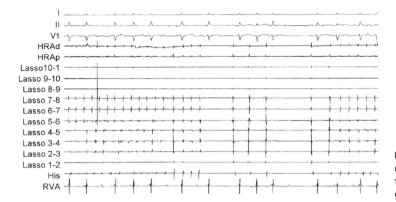

Figure 37.2 Termination and re-initiation of ongoing atrial fibrillation during RF pulse delivery.

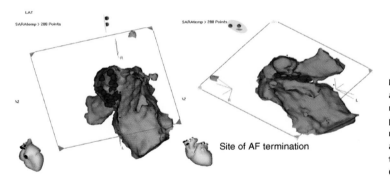

Site of AF termination

Figure 37.3 Site of termination at the crista between the anterior rim of the superior lateral pulmonary vein and the posterior rim of the entrance of the left appendage, as identified on the three-dimensional reconstructed CARTO™ merge map.

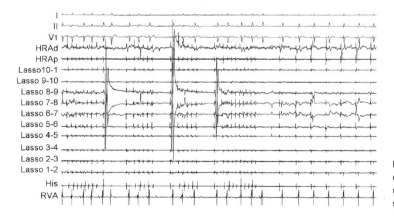

Figure 37.4 During RF pulse delivery at the same site as reported in Figure 37.2, stable sinus rhythm is obtained.

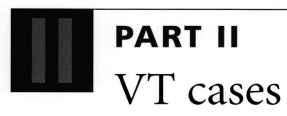

PART II
VT cases

CHAPTER 38

PVC and nonsustained ventricular tachycardia baltion in a child

George Van Hare, MD

Clinical vignette

An 11-year-old male presented with frequent premature ventricular complexes (PVCs), nonsustained ventricular tachycardia, and symptoms of palpitations. The patient also has a history of asthma. His heart was structurally and functionally normal by echocardiogram. He is unable to tolerate beta-blockers because of his asthma. He was referred for ablation.

Electrophysiology study and ablation

The procedure was performed under general anesthesia, using the NavX system. Nonsustained ventricular tachycardia with a left bundle branch morphology was repeatedly induced (Figure 38.1). Activation maps of the right and left ventricles revealed the site of earliest activation to be in the right ventricular outflow tract (Figure 38.2). Application of radiofrequency energy in this location rendered the patient no longer inducible.

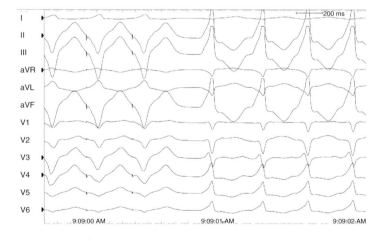

Figure 38.1 Nonsustained ventricular tachycardia was repeatedly inducible with the infusion of isoproterenol, using ventricular burst pacing. A 12-lead ECG shows that it has a left bundle branch block morphology and an inferior frontal plane axis.

Electroanatomical Mapping, 1st edition. Edited by
A. Al-Ahmad, D. Callans, H. Hsia and A. Natale.
© 2008 Blackwell Publishing, ISBN: 9781405157025.

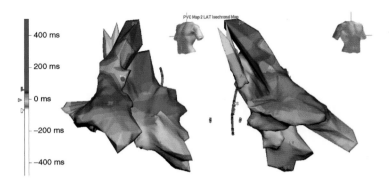

Figure 38.2 Both ventricles are mapped, the right via the tricuspid valve and the left via a retrograde approach to the left ventricle. Isochronal maps of spontaneous uniform PVCs are referenced to the right ventricular apex. The earliest local ventricular activation is in the left lateral aspect of the right ventricular outflow tract.

CHAPTER 39

Electroanatomical mapping for ventricular premature complexes from the right ventricular outflow tract

Henry A. Chen, MD *& Paul J. Wang,* MD

Clinical vignette

A 70-year-old male with a history of nonischemic cardiomyopathy, with a biventricular implantable cardioverter defibrillator (ICD), presented with episodes of weakness and dizziness. He has been found to have multiple ventricular premature complexes (VPCs) consistent with origin from the right ventricular outflow tract on outpatient ECGs (Figure 39.1). A recent coronary catheterization revealed no significant stenosis. After beta-blocker therapy was unable to control his symptoms, he was referred for catheter ablation.

Electrophysiology study and ablation

Baseline electrophysiological characteristics were normal. There was no inducible ventricular or supraventricular tachycardia. The patient had

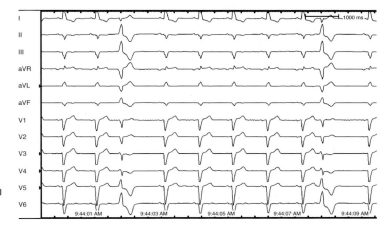

FFigure 39.1 Baseline ECG: spontaneous VPCs had a left bundle branch block type pattern, isoelectric in V4, negative in leads I and aVL, and positive in lead II, III, and aVF

Electroanatomical Mapping, 1st edition. Edited by
A. Al-Ahmad, D. Callans, H. Hsia and A. Natale.
© 2008 Blackwell Publishing, ISBN: 9781405157025.

frequent spontaneous VPCs, which matched his clinical beats on outpatient ECGs. A three-dimensional anatomical shell of the right ventricle and outflow tract was created on the NavX system (Figure 39.2). Pace-mapping and activation mapping of multiple monomorphic ventricular beats were performed. Earliest activation was found in the mid-septal region of the right ventricular outflow tract (Figures 39.3 and 39.4).

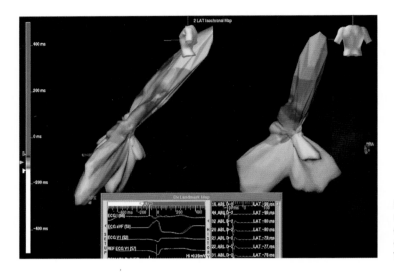

Figure 39.2 Electroanatomical mapping showed the area of earliest right ventricular activation during spontaneous monomorphic VPCs.

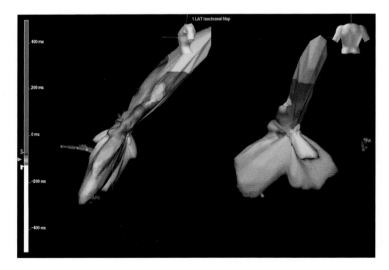

Figure 39.3 Ablation lesions delivered to the site of earliest ventricular activation (yellow, blue, and green dots). Ablation at this area resulted in increased frequency of VPCs at initiation of energy delivery followed by the absence of VPCs during remainder of ablation and during observation period.

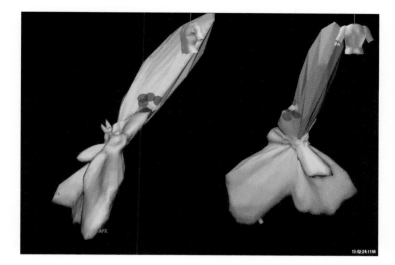

Figure 39.4   Lesion set (brown dots) as "insurance ablations" delivered in rosette pattern around site of ablation of earliest ventricular activation.

CHAPTER 40

Ablation of idiopathic RV ventricular tachycardia in an unusual location using EnSite mapping

David Callans, MD, FACC, FHRS

Clinical vignette

The patient is a 39-year-old man who carried the diagnosis of arrhythmogenic RV dysplasia and had infrequent episodes of rapid ventricular tachycardia (VT) (210 bpm) with exercise. The diagnosis of arrhythmogenic right ventricular dysplasia (ARVD) was made at an outside center 7 years earlier on the basis of VTs originating from the right ventricle with "an abnormal MRI," and an implantable cardioverter defibrillator (ICD) was implanted. Because of drug refractory VT and concern about the accuracy of the underlying diagnosis, an ablation procedure was planned.

Electrophysiology study and ablation

The patient presented to the electrophysiology lab in normal sinus rhythm. The clinical VT morphology (matching previous ICD electrograms) was induced reproducibly with programmed stimulation (Figure 40.1). EnSite noncontact array mapping demonstrated normal-appearing unipolar electrograms throughout the RV and at the site of origin of the VT. Isopotential mapping demonstrated several unique features (Figure 40.2): (1) the

earliest activation was recorded on the endocardial surface preceded the "exit site," defined as the area of diffuse early endocardial activation and the site at which pace-mapping matched the VT morphology; (2) the exit site occurred fairly late compared with the onset of the VT QRS; and (3) although the "channel" of activation prior to the exit site was earlier, an initial R wave on the local unipolar electrogram suggested a deeper (subendocardial?) location of this activation. Ablation at a site within this channel (Figure 40.3), distant from the exit site, resulted in inability to induce the tachycardia. The patient has been well without recurrence for 3 years. The diagnosis of ARVD on the basis of MRI is treacherous and may lack precision in all but the most advanced centers. Endocardial mapping, to determine the presence/absence of low-voltage substrate at the site of origin of the VT, seems to be more reliable. In this case, the diagnosis was refuted by this technique. The directional capabilities of unipolar recordings can be very important for mapping. At the true site of origin of a focal tachycardia, activation spreads away in all directions. This is reflected by qS morphology in the unipolar electrogram. An initial R wave on the unipolar recording indicates spread of activation toward the site of recording; if this site is the earliest endocardial site, this spread of activation must come from deeper layers of the myocardium. Even in what would be considered focal tachycardias, presystolic "channels" of conduction leading to the exit site have been identified.

Electroanatomical Mapping, 1st edition. Edited by A. Al-Ahmad, D. Callans, H. Hsia and A. Natale. © 2008 Blackwell Publishing, ISBN: 9781405157025.

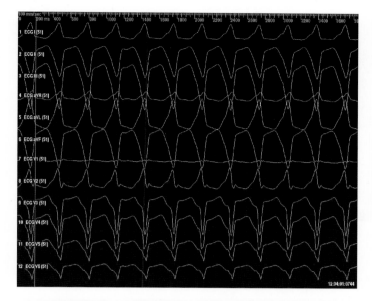

Figure 40.1 Right bundle (with early transition) left, inferior axis VT induced in the electrophysiology lab. Intracardiac electrograms recorded from the ICD matched spontaneous events.

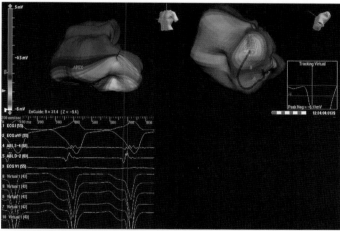

Figure 40.2 The "exit site" demonstrated with isopotential mapping (top) was diffuse; activation here was late compared with the onset of the QRS. An earlier "channel" (below, traced with the gray line) was demonstrated. Unipolar electrograms recorded along the channel had an earlier local activation times, although still after the QRS onset, and had a small initial R wave.

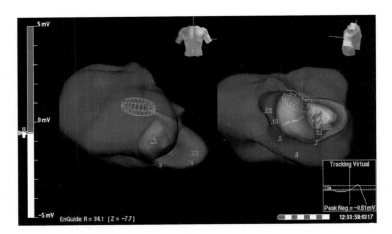

Figure 40.3   A series of ablation lesions placed at the start of the "channel" resulted in elimination of the clinical VT.

CHAPTER 41

Ablation of poorly inducible fascicular ventricular tachycardia

Jason Jacobson, MD

Clinical vignette

A 17-year-old man presented to the emergency department with the sudden onset of palpitations while doing push-ups. A wide-complex tachycardia (WCT) at a rate of 200 bpm was recorded on a 12-lead ECG. Adenosine 12 mg was given without termination of the tachycardia. A 75-J biphasic external cardioversion shock restored sinus rhythm. Figure 41.1 shows the surface 12-lead ECG of the WCT with a right bundle branch block (RBBB), right-superior axis (RBRS) morphology.

Electrophysiology study and ablation

The patient presented to the electrophysiology laboratory in normal sinus rhythm. With isoproterenol infusion, atrial pacing near the clinical tachycardia rate resulted in 1:1 conduction with an RBBB aberrancy similar to the morphology of the clinical tachycardia (Figure 41.2). In addition, AV nodal echo beats were induced with single atrial extrastimuli. However, with programmed stimulation from the right ventricle, a WCT was induced, with ventriculo-atrial Wenckebach conduction pattern consistent with the diagnosis of ventricular tachycardia (VT) (Figure 41.3). The morphology of this VT matched the clinical WCT and was suggestive of a left posterior fascicular VT.

Left ventricular electroanatomical mapping was performed. A Purkinje potential (PP) was recorded at the posterior septum prior to the onset of the QRS in the proximal mapping catheter during VT with a PP fused with a ventricular electrograms in the distal poles (Figure 41.4).

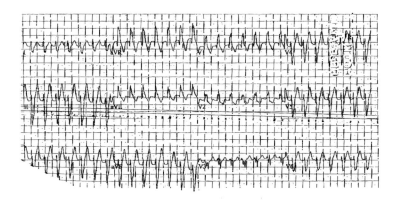

Figure 41.1 Surface 12-lead ECG of the RBB-right-superior (RBRS) QRS axis WCT.

Electroanatomical Mapping, 1st edition. Edited by A. Al-Ahmad, D. Callans, H. Hsia and A. Natale. © 2008 Blackwell Publishing, ISBN: 9781405157025.

Catheter contact in this area terminated the VT and could not be re-initiated. Mechanical pressure with catheter contact in the proximal left posterior fascicle area more basal on the septum induced spontaneous ventricular beats identical to the VT, which were preceded by a PP (Figure 41.5). The areas with the presystolic Purkinje potentials were tagged along the posterior ventricular septum to outline the locations of the left posterior fascicle.

Owing to the inability to re-induce the VT, an anatomic approach to ablation was undertaken. A linear lesion set was created perpendicular to the long axis of the septum, transecting the locations of the left posterior fascicle where catheter-induced beats were seen preceded by a PP (Figure 41.6). The entire ventricle displayed normal voltage (>1.5 mV). After ablation, the frontal plane axis on the surface ECG changed to a more rightward, inferior axis (Figure 41.7), consistent with an iatrogenic left posterior fascicular block.

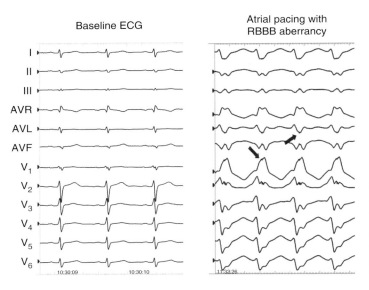

Figure 41.2 Atrial pacing at 250 ms on isoproterenol. Note the right bundle branch block aberrancy and right superior frontal axis, similar to that of the clinical RBBB tachycardia. The arrows indicate the atrial pacing stimulus artifacts with a long stimulus-to-QRS interval.

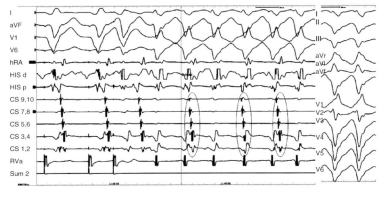

Figure 41.3 Induction of VT with a single ventricular extra-stimulus. The tracing consisted of surface leads I, aVf, V1, and V6, with intracardiac recordings of high right atrium (HRA), His recordings (His), coronary sinus (CS), and right ventricle (RV). The circles identified atrial electrograms in the CS recordings that demonstrated ventriculo-atrial dissociation. The tracing on the right displays the full 12-lead ECG of the VT.

Figure 41.4 Left ventricular mapping with septal electrogram recordings during VT. The intracardiac recordings were similar to that of Figure 41.3 with the additional mapping catheter recordings (CARTO™). Note the Purkinje potentials (circles and arrows) that precede the onset of QRS. Ventricular myocardial potentials in the mapping catheter, with the proximal PPs preceding the distal PPs.

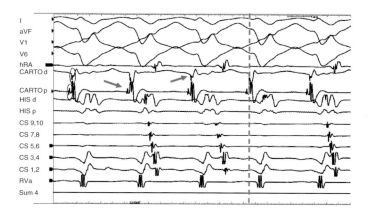

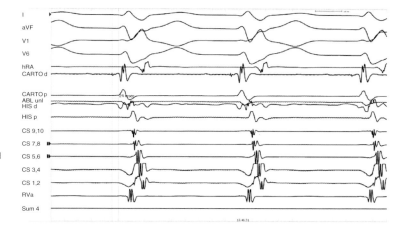

Figure 41.5 Catheter-induced ventricular beats from the left posterior fascicle. The PP precedes the QRS by 24 ms. QRS morphology matches the VT.

Figure 41.6 Right anterior oblique (RAO-left) and modified posteroanterior (PA-right) views of the linear ablation lesion (red dots) set on CARTO™. The ablation line transected the location of the left posterior fascicle. For better illustration, a white dot line was superimposed over the electroanatomic maps to represent the linear ablation lesion.

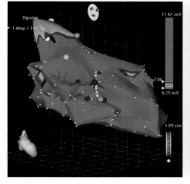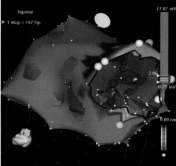

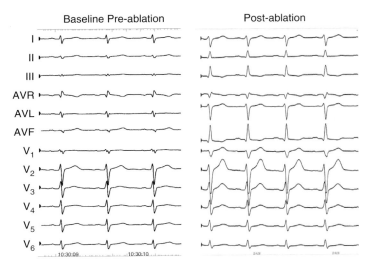

Figure 41.7   A 12-lead ECG of sinus rhythm after completion of the linear ablation lesion set. Note that the frontal axis has shifted to the right compared with the baseline ECG, consistent with a newly induced left posterior fascicular conduction delay.

CHAPTER 42

Electroanatomic mapping for left anterior fascicular ventricular tachycardia

David Callans, MD, FACC, FHRS

Clinical vignette

A 43-year-old man with exercise-induced palpitations was referred for catheter ablation of presumed idiopathic ventricular tachycardia (VT). At peak exercise, he had sudden increase in heart rate to 160/min, which eventually resolved with rest. There was no history of syncope or presyncope. An echocardiogram was normal. An outside electrophysiologic study, where programmed stimulation was performed but isoproterenol was not infused, did not reproduce the tachycardia.

Electrophysiology study and ablation

On 10 mcg/min of isoproterenol, a right-bundle-right-inferior (RBRI) VT was induced with burst ventricular pacing (Figure 42.1). Pacing the atrium during sinus rhythm at the tachycardia cycle length did not result in right bundle branch block (RBBB) aberration. Pacing from the LV consistently resulted in VT termination.

Mapping ensued with pace-mapping during sinus rhythm. Because of the tachycardia

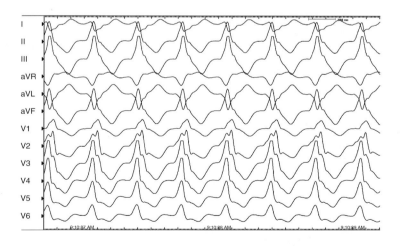

Figure 42.1 VT induced with burst ventricular pacing on isoproterenol, matching the clinical RBRI morphology and a cycle length of 360 ms.

Electroanatomical Mapping, 1st edition. Edited by
A. Al-Ahmad, D. Callans, H. Hsia and A. Natale.
© 2008 Blackwell Publishing, ISBN: 9781405157025.

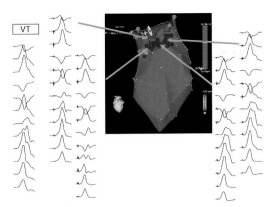

morphology and pace-map location, a site of origin from the left anterior fascicle was considered (Figure 42.2); however, fascicular potentials were not observed at good pace-map sites during sinus rhythm or during VT.

Several ablations were delivered to this area, usually resulting in slow ectopy matching the VT morphology during radiofrequency. At the end of the study, no further VT was initiated with programmed stimulation and high-dose isoproterenol (Figure 42.3).

Figure 42.2 Pace-mapping for the clinical VT morphology, and the creation of the eventual lesion set near the left anterior fascicle.

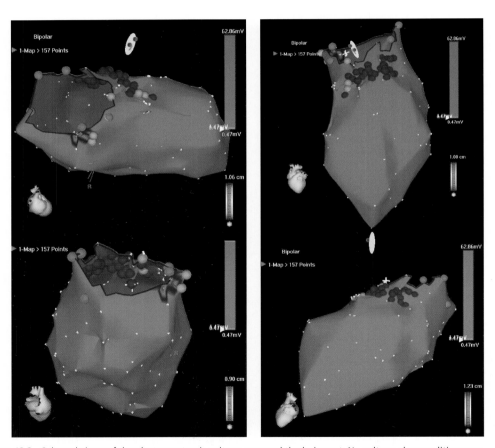

Figure 42.3 Selected views of the electroanatomic voltage map and the lesion set. No voltage abnormalities were observed, and the LV was normal in size.

CHAPTER 43

Left ventricular tachycardia originating in basal diverticulum

Sumeet K. Mainigi, MD

Clinical vignette

The patient is a 75-year-old woman with long-standing palpitations maintained on a beta-blocker. Four months prior to the present admission, she developed sustained, rapid palpitations and was evaluated in the emergency room. She was found to have a wide-complex tachycardia that terminated spontaneously. Her beta-blocker was increased and she was discharged. One week prior to admission, she developed severe palpitations and near syncope. She was found to be in a wide-complex tachycardia (Figure 43.1). She was given amiodarone without change and received a 200-J shock, which terminated the arrhythmia. A subsequent echocardiogram, stress test, and cardiac catheterization demonstrated normal cardiac function and no significant coronary artery disease, although a focal structural abnormality was seen (Figure 43.2).

Electrophysiology study and ablation

Electroanatomic mapping of the left ventricle demonstrated a small apical scar and a diverticulum along the anterolateral wall with scar at its apex. An intracardiac echocardiogram confirmed the presence of diverticulum (Figure 43.3). Concealed entrainment with a long stimulus-to-QRS interval was demonstrated from multiple areas in the apex of the outpouching, consistent with entrance sites (Figures 43.4 and 43.5). An electroanatomic

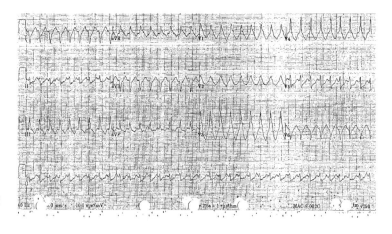

Figure 43.1 A 12-lead electrocardiogram of clinically observed ventricular tachycardia. The EKG demonstrated a right-bundle-right-inferior (RBRI) QRS axis, suggesting a likely exit site along the anterolateral wall of the left ventricle.

Electroanatomical Mapping, 1st edition. Edited by
A. Al-Ahmad, D. Callans, H. Hsia and A. Natale.
© 2008 Blackwell Publishing, ISBN: 9781405157025.

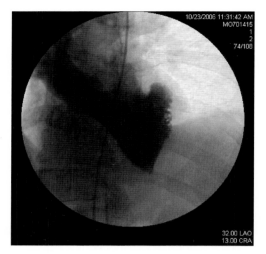

Figure 43.2 Left ventriculogram in left anterior oblique (LAO) view demonstrates an outpouching along the anterolateral wall.

activation map was created of the diverticulum and the earliest site of activation at which concealed entrainment was demonstrated was targeted (Figures 43.6 and 43.7). The arrhythmia terminated 22 s into the radiofrequency lesion at this location (Figure 43.8).

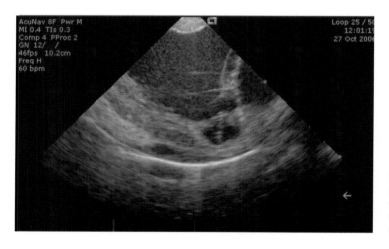

Figure 43.3 The mapping catheter was advanced into the diverticulum. Intracardiac echocardiography demonstrating ablation catheter in diverticulum.

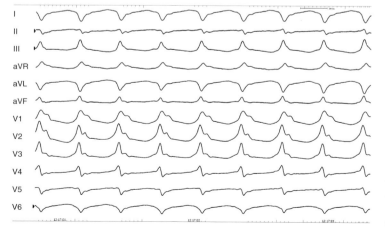

Figure 43.4 The clinically observed ventricular tachycardia was induced with programmed stimulation from the right ventricular apex and more easily from the left ventricular diverticulum. The tachycardia was hemodynamically tolerated, allowing mapping.

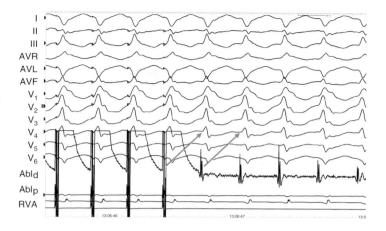

Figure 43.5   Concealed entrainment was demonstrated at multiple distal sites within the diverticulum. At this site, the postpacing interval (PPI) equals the VT cycle length, with a long stimulus-to-QRS interval (Stim–QRS) that equals the electrogram-to-QRS interval (Egm–QRS), consistent with an entrance site.

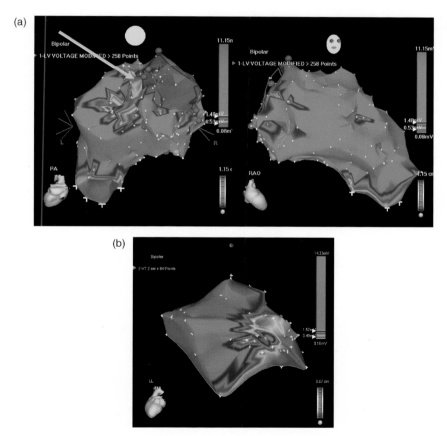

Figure 43.6   (a) Posterior and right anterior oblique views of a left ventricle voltage map created in sinus rhythm demonstrate an apical area of scar (red) and an area of lower voltage along the anterolateral wall at the base of the diverticulum (yellow arrow). (b) A second map was created of the diverticulum. A left lateral view of the diverticular voltage map obtained during ventricular tachycardia demonstrates scar at the apex of outpouching.

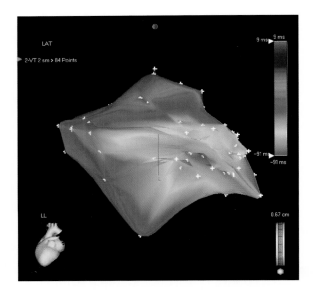

Figure 43.7   Left lateral view activation map of ventricular tachycardia, focusing primarily on diverticulum shown in Figure 43.6B. The earliest activation is depicted in red, and the blue/purple colored area represents late activation.

(a)

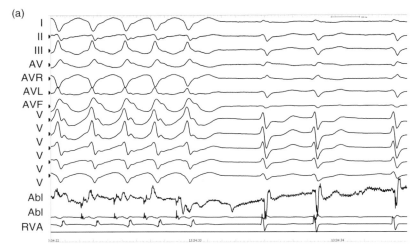

(b)

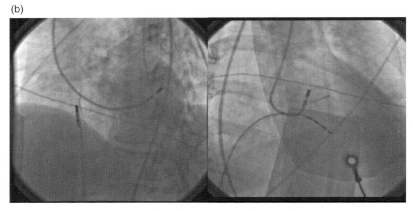

Figure 43.8   (a) Termination of tachycardia 22 s into the ablation lesion. (b) LAO and RAO fluoroscopic images at the site of termination.

CHAPTER 44

PVC originating near aortic cusps

Sumeet K. Mainigi, MD

Clinical vignette

The patient is a 59-year-old man with palpitations. During a colonoscopy, he demonstrated frequent nonsustained ventricular tachycardia and frequent premature ventricular complexes (PVCs) of the same morphology (Figure 44.1). Physical examination and echocardiogram were unremarkable.

Electrophysiology study and ablation

A mapping catheter was advanced into the right ventricular outflow tract (RVOT). An electroanatomic activation map was created of the RVOT and demonstrated diffuse posteroseptal activation (Figure 44.2). Pace-mapping was performed in the RVOT but failed to demonstrate a suitable match. The catheter was advanced retrograde into the left ventricular outflow tract and aortic cusp region, and a second activation map was created (Figure 44.3). Activation mapping demonstrated that the RVOT was late relative to the left outflow/aortic cusp region. The earliest activation site was between the left and right aortic cusps. Pace-mapping at this site demonstrated a good match to the clinical PVC (Figure 44.4). A radiofrequency lesion at this site terminated the arrhythmia (Figure 44.5).

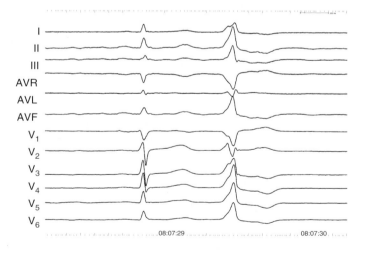

Figure 44.1 Frequent PVCs were observed at rest. All PVCs have an identical left bundle branch block left-inferior (LBLI) QRS axis morphology, suggesting an outflow tract origin. The PVC QRS has an early precordial transition, suggesting a left ventricular outflow tract origin.

Electroanatomical Mapping, 1st edition. Edited by
A. Al-Ahmad, D. Callans, H. Hsia and A. Natale.
© 2008 Blackwell Publishing, ISBN: 9781405157025.

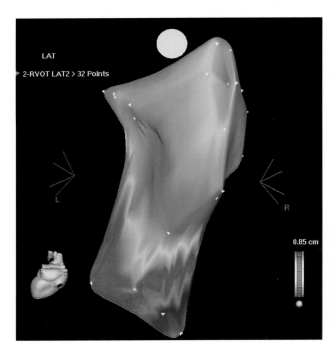

Figure 44.2 Electroanatomic mapping of the right ventricular outflow tract (RVOT) in posterior-anterior (PA) view. Activation mapping of the clinical PVC demonstrates diffuse activation along the posteroseptal aspect of the right ventricular outflow tract. The earliest activation is depicted by red, and the blue/purple colored area represents late activation.

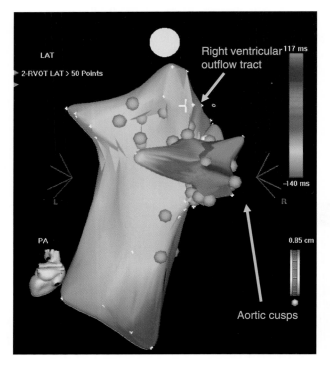

Figure 44.3 Limited map of aortic cusps and the left ventricular outflow tract in a PA view demonstrates earlier activation (red) relative to the right ventricular outflow tract. The aortic cusps are posterior and inferior to the top of the RVOT at the level of the pulmonary valve.

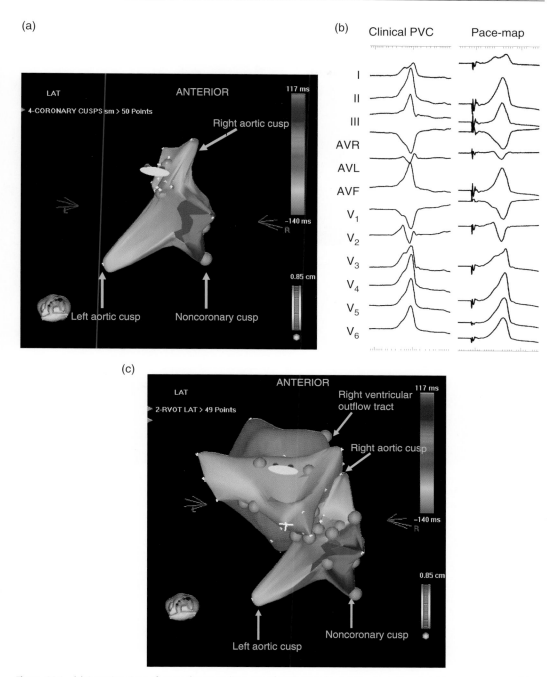

Figure 44.4 (a) Superior view of cusps shows earliest site of activation (red) between left and right coronary cusps. (b) The pace-map at the earliest site (see gray dot in Figure 44.5). (c) A superior view shows the relationship of the left ventricular cusps and right ventricular outflow tract.

(a)

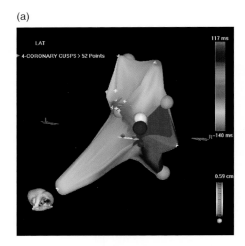

(b)

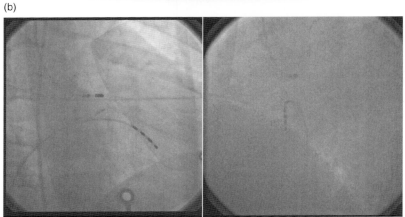

Figure 44.5   (a) A superior view of the CARTO™ activation map of the aortic cusps showing the site of the successful ablation lesion that terminated the PVC. The gray dot is the site of the best pace-map in Figure 44.4b. (b) Right anterior oblique (RAO) (left) and left anterior oblique (LAO) (right) fluoroscopic images at successful ablation site.

CHAPTER 45

Right ventricular outflow tachycardia

Kevin Makati, MD *& N. A. Mark Estes III,* MD

Clinical vignette

A 43-year-old with no significant past medical history presented with symptomatic premature ventricular contractions (PVCs). A cardiac evaluation revealed normal right and left ventricular function. A stress test showed no ischemia. A Holter monitor showed a high frequency of monomorphic nonsustained ventricular tachycardia (VT). A 12-lead ECG revealed PVCs with an origin consistent with the right ventricular outflow tract (Figure 45.1).

Electrophysiology study and ablation

Spontaneous PVCs were mapped using a combination of pace-mapping and activation mapping with the CARTO™ system. At the site of successful ablation, a perfect pace-map was obtained. Lesion delivery was successful in eliminating spontaneous PVCs (Figure 45.2).

Right ventricular outflow tachycardia accounts for approximately 10% of the VTs. The 12-lead

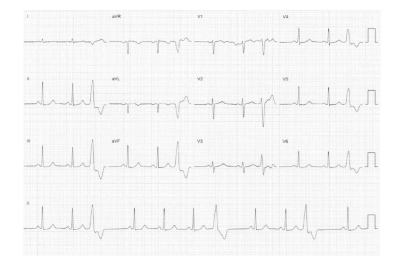

Figure 45.1 A 12-lead electrocardiogram shows PVCs of left bundle branch block morphology with a transition point in precordial lead V3, inferior frontal plane axis, and negative limb lead I, consistent with an anteroseptal right ventricular outflow tract origin.

Electroanatomical Mapping, 1st edition. Edited by
A. Al-Ahmad, D. Callans, H. Hsia and A. Natale.
© 2008 Blackwell Publishing, ISBN: 9781405157025.

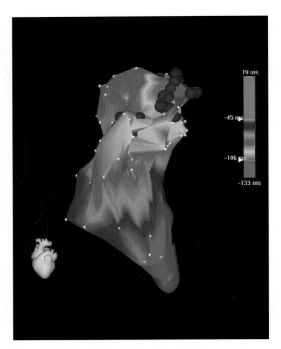

Figure 45.2 The electroanatomical activation map shows a left anterior oblique (LAO) projection of the right ventricle. The area of earliest activation is colored in red and latest activation in purple with a gradient of activation times in between. The red spheres indicate ablation points.

electrocardiogram can be useful in approximating the location of the PVCs. Although previous studies have suggested that pace-mapping may be more precise in locating the site of origin compared with activation mapping for idiopathic focal VTs, a more recent investigation has shown a comparable efficacy between pace-mapping and activation mapping with the electroanatomic mapping system.

CHAPTER 46

Right ventricular outflow tract polymorphic ventricular tachycardia

Luis C. Sáenz, MD, *Miguel A. Vacca,* MD, MSc, *& Andrea Natale,* MD, FACC, FHRS

Clinical vignette

A 45-year-old woman presented with recurrent syncope preceded by palpitations that occurred both with exercise as well as occasionally at rest in the supine position. She had no significant prior medical history or familial history of sudden death. A Holter showed frequent and monomorphic premature ventricular complexes (PVCs), and she was treated with beta-adrenergic-blockers. The echocardiogram was normal, and a signal-averaged EKG was normal. Despite beta-blockers, she had recurrence of the syncope. She was hospitalized on a telemetry unit where an EKG during symptoms was recorded (Figure 46.1). Therefore, the origin of the episodes of syncope was considered as probably related to polymorphic ventricular tachycardia (VT) triggered by PVC from the right ventricular

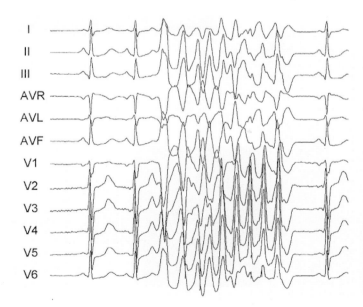

Figure 46.1 EKG showing a short polymorphic VT triggered by PVC with a short coupling interval. The morphology of the PVC suggests origin on the superior and posterior aspect of the RVOT.

Electroanatomical Mapping, 1st edition. Edited by A. Al-Ahmad, D. Callans, H. Hsia and A. Natale.
© 2008 Blackwell Publishing, ISBN: 9781405157025.

outflow tract (RVOT). The patient underwent VT ablation.

Electrophysiology study and ablation

The patient was brought to the electrophysiology laboratory. Electroanatomical mapping of the spontaneous PVCs using the CARTO™ system was employed. The area of early activation (about −30 ms from the QRS onset) was close to the area of best pace-map (Figure 46.2). After the initial applications, the PVC frequency decreased significantly but some PVCs with similar EKG morphology remained. Because of this, the radiofrequency (RF) applications were extended through the best pace-map zone. An episode of nonsustained polymorphic VT was induced during the RF application, as shown in Figure 46.3. After 10 months of follow-up free of medications, the patient has not shown any PVC or VT recurrence.

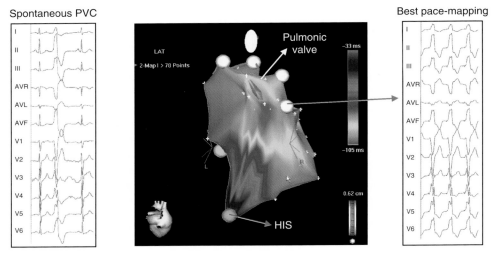

Figure 46.2 Electroanatomical reconstruction of the RVOT showing the activation mapping from a right posterior oblique (RPO) view. The map suggests a focal arrhythmia with the earliest activation area over the superior and posterior aspect of the RVOT. The best pace-map was obtained from an area 4 mm away from the site of earliest activation.

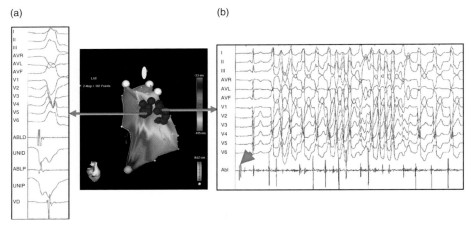

Figure 46.3 Panel (a) Electroanatomical reconstruction of the RVOT from the same view as Figure 46.2. The ablation lesions were initially applied over the earliest CARTO™ zone where the obtained electrogram-to-QRS interval was 30 ms. The unipolar electrogram 1 (UNI 1) showed an excellent QS pattern with a presystolic local activation. Panel (b) shows a run of pleomorphic VT induced during RF application.

CHAPTER 47

Left aortic cusp ventricular tachycardia

John Sussman, MD

Clinical vignette

A 51-year-old male reported episodic palpitations for 2 years. Baseline ECG revealed frequent premature ventricular complexes (PVCs). A treadmill stress test was performed, and he developed sustained monomorphic ventricular tachycardia (VT) (Figure 47.1).

Electrophysiology study and ablation

Spontaneous VT with morphology similar to the clinical arrhythmia was seen (Figure 47.2). Differences in axis were noted, possibly relating to slightly different lead position or posture. Sinus rhythm voltage maps of the right and left ventricles

were created, revealing grossly normal endocardial voltages in both right and left ventricles (Figure 47.3). Pace-maps from both the right ventricular outflow tract and left ventricular outflow tract were a poor match for the VT. The aortic cusps were subsequently mapped, and their anatomic locations delineated just below the level of the right ventricular outflow tract (Figure 47.4). Local activation in the left coronary cusp was 33 ms pre-QRS, and pace-maps were a perfect match for the VT. Both electroanatomic mapping (Figure 47.5) and angiography (Figure 47.6) were performed to confirm a safe distance between the left main coronary artery and the ablation site in the left coronary cusp. Ablation was performed, rendering the VT noninducible. No complications were seen relating to this ablation site.

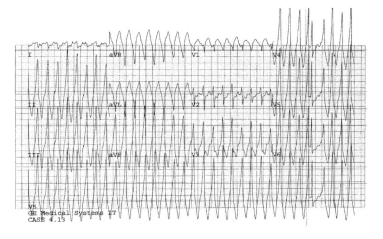

Figure 47.1 Electrocardiogram showing ventricular tachycardia during stress testing. The VT has a left bundle branch block-right-inferior (LBRI) QRS morphology with an early precordial transition, suggestive of a left ventricular outflow tract (LVOT) origin.

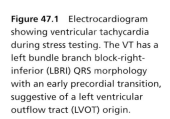

Electroanatomical Mapping, 1st edition. Edited by A. Al-Ahmad, D. Callans, H. Hsia and A. Natale. © 2008 Blackwell Publishing, ISBN: 9781405157025.

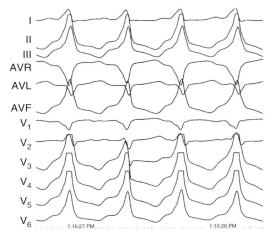

Figure 47.2 Electrocardiogram of a left bundle branch block-left-inferior (LBLI) QRS morphology ventricular tachycardia during procedure; note the difference in lead I and an earlier precordial transition.

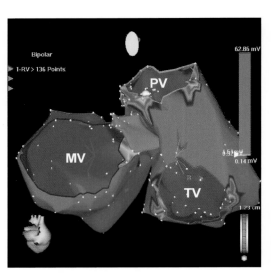

Figure 47.4 Posteroanterior view of left ventricle, right ventricle, and aortic cusps (green). Noted the aortic cusp is posterior to the right ventricular outflow tract and inferior to the pulmonic valve. MV: mitral valve; TV: tricuspid valve; and PV: pulmonic valve.

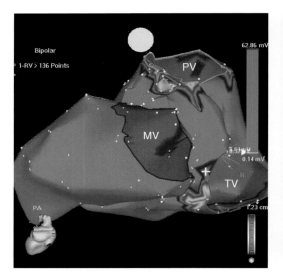

Figure 47.3 Posteroanterior view of left and right ventricular voltage maps in sinus rhythm. The purple colored area represents normal endocardium (amplitude ≥1.5 mV), and dense scar is depicted as red (amplitude <0.5 mV). The border zone (amplitude 0.5–1.5 mV) is defined as areas with the intermediate color gradient. MV: mitral valve; TV: tricuspid valve; and PV: pulmonic valve.

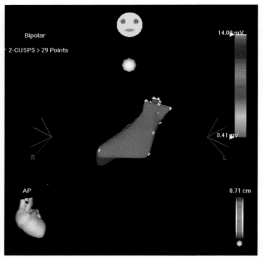

Figure 47.5 CARTO™ map of aortic cusps with white spot representing ostium of left main coronary artery. The distance between the left main coronary artery ostium and the aortic cusp was approximately 1 cm.

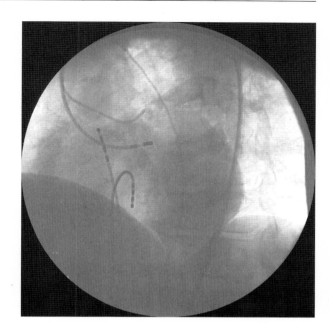

Figure 47.6   Left anterior oblique fluoroscopy showing ablation catheter in left coronary cusp and JL4 catheter engaged in left main coronary artery.

CHAPTER 48

Ventricular tachycardia in patient with tetralogy of Fallot

Dajoon Anh, MD *Amin Al-Ahmad,* MD *& Henry Hsia,* MD

Clinical vignette

A 38-year-old male with a history of tetralogy of Fallot presented with ventricular tachycardia (VT) (cycle length of 440 ms) producing near syncope. He had previously undergone a right ventricular outflow aneurysmectomy and homograft replacement of the pulmonary valve. An echocardiogram (ECG) showed moderate RV systolic dysfunction accompanied by moderate pulmonary regurgitation. The sinus rhythm ECG was significant for right bundle branch block with a QRS duration of 215 ms (Figure 48.1).

Electrophysiology study and ablation

At electrophysiology study, a right bundle right inferior ventricular tachycardia with cycle length of 440 ms reproducing the clinical arrhythmia was induced (Figure 48.2). Sinus voltage map of the RV showed extensive areas of dense scar at superior aspects of the RV outflow tract (Figures 48.3 and 48.4), where late potentials with significant delay were noted (Figure 48.1). Pacing at these sites during VT showed concealed entrainment with identical stimulus-to-QRS (stim–QRS) and EGM–QRS

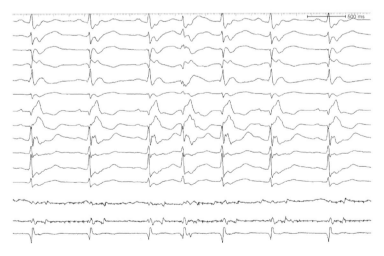

Figure 48.1 The surface ECG during atrial rhythm is shown, along with intracardiac electrograms from the ablation catheter positioned at the right ventricular outflow tract. The ECG shows sinus rhythm with premature atrial complexes with a wide (215 ms) right bundle branch block QRS morphology. The local intracardiac recording at the right ventricular outflow tract shows low-amplitude far-field EGM followed by late potentials (arrows) during sinus rhythm, indicating the presence of slowly conducting myocardium within the scar.

Electroanatomical Mapping, 1st edition. Edited by
A. Al-Ahmad, D. Callans, H. Hsia and A. Natale.
© 2008 Blackwell Publishing, ISBN: 9781405157025.

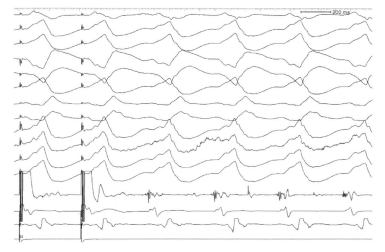

Figure 48.2 Pacing from the right ventricular outflow tract during ventricular tachycardia (right-bundle-right-inferior axis) resulted in concealed entrainment with postpacing interval within 10 ms of the tachycardia cycle length. This site also showed matching stimulus–QRS and EGM–QRS intervals. Ablation performed at this site during tachycardia terminated the arrhythmia in less than 1.0 s (not shown).

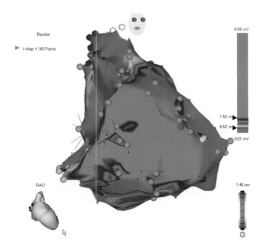

Figure 48.3 Sinus rhythm voltage map of the right ventricle in the right anterior oblique view. Myocardial scar (defined by EGM amplitude <0.5 mV) is outlined with red color. Normal tissue (EGM voltage >1.5 mV) is depicted in purple, and the intervening colors denote border zone tissue (defined by EGM amplitude between 0.5 mV and 1.5 mV).

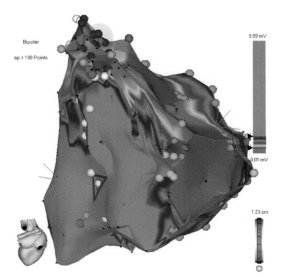

Figure 48.4 Sinus rhythm voltage map of the right ventricle in the posterior view. The posterior right ventricular outflow tract showed scarred myocardium, with some areas demonstrating the absence of local electrograms despite good catheter contact (gray circles). Concealed entrainment and matching stimulus–QRS and EGM–QRS intervals was demonstrated at the edge of the abnormal tissue (white circle). A linear line of lesions from the normal myocardium to the pulmonary valve was constructed starting from the site marked with the white circle. The ventricular tachycardia was no longer inducible after the ablation.

intervals (Figure 48.2). Deployment of a single radiofrequency lesion in this area terminated VT. A line of radiofrequency lesions starting from this site extending inferior to the edge of the scar and superior to the pulmonic valve (Figure 48.4) rendered the VT noninducible.

CHAPTER 49

Ventricular tachycardia in a patient with cardiac sarcoid

Rupa Bala, MD *& David J. Callans,* MD, FACC, FHRS

Clinical vignette

A 50-year-old white female with a history of pulmonary and cardiac sarcoidosis presented with recurrent ventricular tachycardia (VT) refractory to medications.

Electrophysiology study and ablation

An electroanatomical map of the left ventricular endocardium was created using the three-dimensional CARTO™ system. Electrophysiology study induced VT with a right bundle morphology and a right superior axis (RBRS) (Figure 49.1). A voltage map of the LV endocardium revealed no evidence of scar (Figure 49.2). Thus, the epicardial space was accessed and a voltage map of the LV epicardium was created. A large lateral epicardial scar was noted and good pace-maps were found in the basal inferolateral wall (Figure 49.3). Limited activation and entrainment mapping were performed in VT given hemodynamic instability. High-output pacing was performed to assess for diaphragmatic capture. Coronary angiography was performed and radiofrequency lesions were delivered at sites with good pace maps with a 4-mm-tip Navistar catheter. Post-RFA, programmed stimulation was performed and the clinical tachycardia could not be induced.

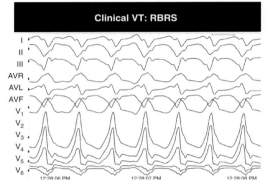

Figure 49.1 Clinical VT: Right bundle, right superior axis (RBRS) VT.

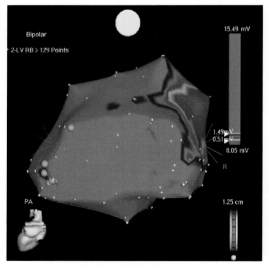

Figure 49.2 Voltage map of LV endocardium created by three-dimensional CARTO™ system with no evidence of endocardial scar. The low-voltage area to the right of the map marks the mitral valve annulus.

Electroanatomical Mapping, 1st edition. Edited by A. Al-Ahmad, D. Callans, H. Hsia and A. Natale.
© 2008 Blackwell Publishing, ISBN: 9781405157025.

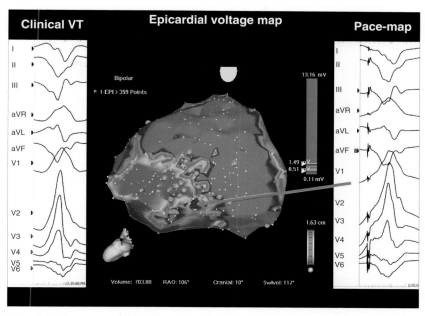

Figure 49.3   Epicardial voltage map and site of best pace-map approximating clinical right bundle VT are shown. RF lesions were given in this area and are marked by the maroon tags.

CHAPTER 50

Ventricular tachycardia in an area of left ventricular noncompaction

John Sussman, MD

Clinical vignette

A 50-year-old female complained of palpitations. Cardiac monitoring revealed premature ventricular complexes (PVCs) and nonsustained ventricular tachycardia (NSVT). Cardiac evaluation was otherwise normal. Two years later, she was admitted to another institution with long runs of NSVT, with a right bundle branch block (RBBB), right inferior axis morphology. At electrophysiology study, two RBBB-type VTs were induced, one with left inferior axis, ablated at the aorto-mitral continuity, and the other with right inferior axis, unsuccessfully ablated in the superolateral left ventricle. She continued to have frequent PVCs and symptomatic episodes of ventricular tachycardia

(VT) (Figure 50.1), and a repeat ablation was performed.

Electrophysiology study and ablation

Frequent spontaneous episodes of VT matching the clinical arrhythmia were seen. Voltage mapping revealed small areas of diminished voltage in the basal anterolateral and basal anteroseptal LV (Figure 50.2). Activation mapping revealed a broad area of early activation in the anterolateral LV (Figure 50.3). Ablation at the site of earliest activation terminated the VT, but it recurred roughly 10 min later with a slightly different morphology, including loss of the small R wave in lead I.

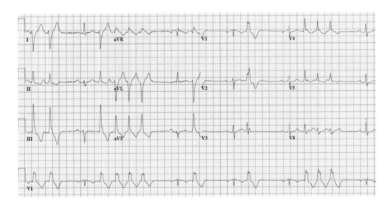

Figure 50.1 The 12-lead electrocardiogram showing spontaneous nonsustained ventricular tachycardia with a right-bundle-right-inferior (RBRI) QRS morphology.

Electroanatomical Mapping, 1st edition. Edited by
A. Al-Ahmad, D. Callans, H. Hsia and A. Natale.
© 2008 Blackwell Publishing, ISBN: 9781405157025.

Intracardiac echo was performed, and revealed an area of noncompacted myocardium with scar near the epicardial surface underlying the anterolateral papillary muscle (Figure 50.4). The catheter was advanced deep into this area. Electroanatomic mapping showed an area with earlier activation jutting out from the left ventricular cavity into the noncompacted myocardium (Figure 50.5a). This area also had lower endocardial voltage (Figure 50.5b). Ablation at this area successfully terminated the VT and rendered it noninducible.

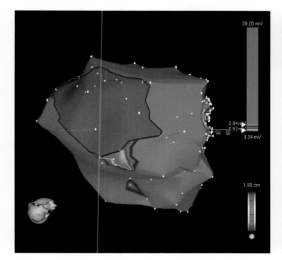

Figure 50.2 Superior view of left ventricular voltage map, showing small areas of decreased voltage and anteroseptum and anterolateral wall.

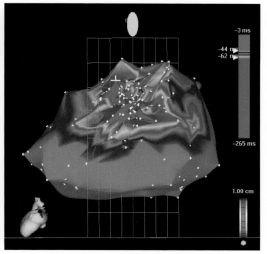

Figure 50.3 Left lateral view of left ventricular activation map, showing diffuse area of early activation. The early activation is depicted as red while purple/blue representing late activation.

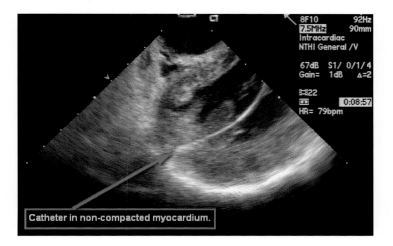

Figure 50.4 Intracardiac echocardiography revealing noncompacted myocardium, with ablation catheter advanced deeply into area of noncompaction.

Catheter in non-compacted myocardium.

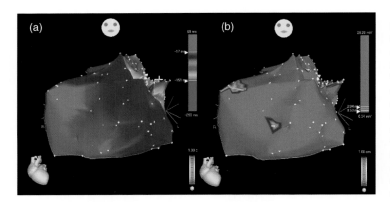

Figure 50.5   (a) Anteroposterior (AP) view of left ventricular activation map. Area of noncompaction is represented by the outpouching of the basal anterolateral wall. The earliest endocardial activation was represented by red overlying the area of noncompaction. (b) AP view of left ventricular voltage map with the area of noncompaction showing lower endocardial voltage than the rest of the LV.

CHAPTER 51

Ventricular tachycardia in a patient with arrhythmogenic right ventricular dysplasia

Rupa Bala, MD

Clinical vignette

The patient is a 53-year-old white male with a history of arrhythmogenic right ventricular dysplasia (ARVD) who was transferred from an outside hospital with palpitations, presyncope, and left bundle morphology ventricular tachycardia (Figure 51.1) for electrophysiology study and ablation.

Electrophysiology study and ablation

An electroanatomical map of the right ventricular endocardium in normal sinus rhythm was created using the three-dimensional CARTO™ system and revealed extensive peri-valvular scar adjacent to the tricuspid valve and extended to the septum and right ventricular outflow tract (RVOT) (Figure 51.2). The apex was spared. Entrainment mapping was used to identify a large, marcoreentrant circuit with an exit site at the RV free wall near the superior aspect of the tricuspid valve annulus (Figure 51.3). RF lesions were given at an isthmus site with tachycardia termination. A linear lesion was extended to the tricuspid valve annulus (Figure 51.4).

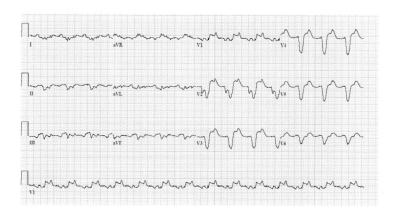

Figure 51.1 Left bundle morphology ventricular tachycardia.

Electroanatomical Mapping, 1st edition. Edited by
A. Al-Ahmad, D. Callans, H. Hsia and A. Natale.
© 2008 Blackwell Publishing, ISBN: 9781405157025.

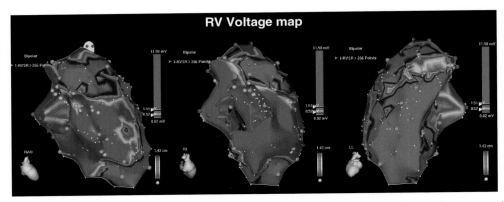

Figure 51.2   Voltage maps of RV endocardium revealing peri-valvular scar extending to the inferior wall, septum, and RVOT, but sparing the RV apex.

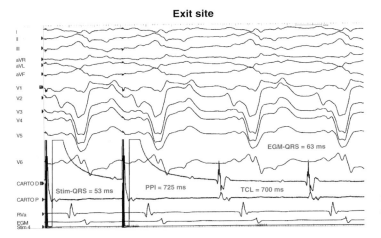

Figure 51.3   Entrainment mapping at exit site of clinical left bundle, left inferior (LBLI) axis VT.

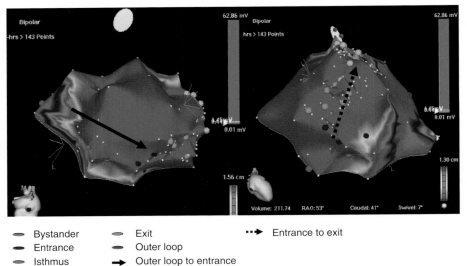

- ⬤ Bystander
- ⬤ Entrance
- ⬤ Isthmus
- ⬤ Exit
- ⬤ Outer loop
- ➡ Outer loop to entrance
- ┅▶ Entrance to exit

Figure 51.4   A large, macroreentrant circuit was identified with entrainment mapping. The entrances through exit sites are shown along the RV free wall adjacent to the tricuspid annulus. Scar was defined as RV endocardial voltage less than 1.5 mV.

CHAPTER 52

Electroanatomical mapping for arrhythmogenic right ventricular dysplasia

Henry Hsia, MD

Clinical vignette

A 42-year-old woman was presented with sustained palpitations. She was found to be in a wide-complex tachycardia (WCT) at ~187 bpm and required cardioversion to restore sinus rhythm (Figure 52.1).

A cardiac catheterization revealed noncritical coronary artery disease. An echocardiogram showed a dilated right ventricular with severe hypokinesis. A diffusely hypokinetic left ventricle was noted with an ejection fraction of approximately 25%.

She underwent a cardiac MRI that demonstrated focal thinning and wall motion abnormalities at multiple areas, especially within the right

ventricular outflow tract (Figure 52.2). A diagnosis of arrhythmogenic right ventricular dysplasia with biventricular involvement was made.

The patient developed recurrent sustained monomorphic ventricular tachycardia (VT) and underwent amiodarone loading.

Electrophysiology study and ablation

Despite aggressive programmed stimulation, no sustained VT was induced. Only frequent spontaneous premature ventricular contractions (PVC) and nonsustained arrhythmia were observed.

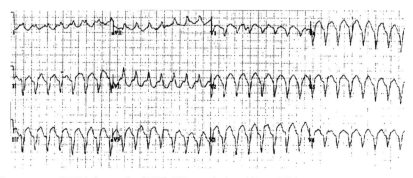

Figure 52.1 Spontaneous LBBB-left-superior (LBLS) QRS morphology VT at ~187 bpm.

Electroanatomical Mapping, 1st edition. Edited by
A. Al-Ahmad, D. Callans, H. Hsia and A. Natale.
© 2008 Blackwell Publishing, ISBN: 9781405157025.

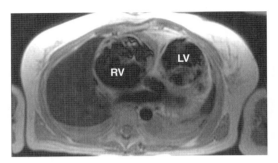

Figure 52.2 Chest MRI showing a dilated, thin right ventricle (RV) and a somewhat enlarged left ventricle (LV).

Despite noninducibility of patient's clinical VT, the potential VT circuit isthmus was identified by selective pacing within conducting channels, based on detailed characterization of the electroanatomic substrate (Figures 52.3–52.5).

Radiofrequency ablation was performed with linear lesions that transected the potential VT circuit. She underwent implantation of a defibrillator. The patient has been clinically stable without recurrent VT.

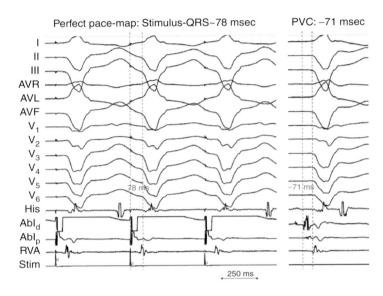

Figure 52.3 Selective pace-mapping based on endocardial voltage characteristics: perfect pace-map with long stim–QRS intervals (78 ms) that equals to the EGM–QRS (71 ms) during spontaneous PVCs.

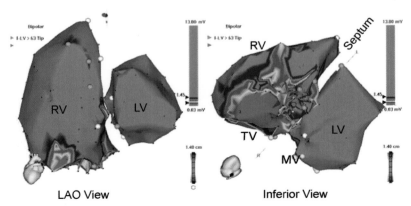

Figure 52.4 Electroanatomic voltage map of both right ventricle (RV) and left ventricle (LV) during sinus rhythm in multiple views shows a normal LV with a markedly dilated RV. Purple colored areas represent normal endocardium (amplitude ≥1.8 mV) while dense scar depicted as red (amplitude <0.5 mV). The border zone (amplitude 0.5–1.8 mV) is defined as areas with the color gradient between red and purple. A large inferior endocardial scar at RV base was present. The tricuspid valve (TV) and mitral valve (MV) annuli are depicted to define the ventricular base.

Figure 52.5 Electroanatomical mapping showed a large inferior-basal RV scar. With high-density endocardial recordings to create a substrate map, a potential "conducting channel" was identified that extended from the dense scar (red) through the border zone into the normal endocardium (purple). The "channel" had a higher bipolar voltage signals than that of the surrounding tissues. Pace-mapping within the channel resulted in a perfectly matched paced QRS compared to the spontaneous VT, with progressively longer stimulus–QRS intervals deeper into the scar.

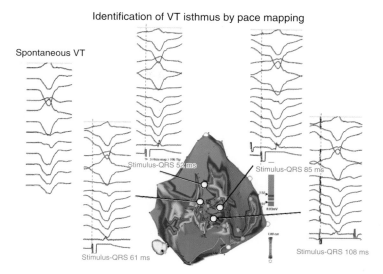

Identification of VT isthmus by pace mapping

Spontaneous VT

Stimulus-QRS 52 ms

Stimulus-QRS 85 ms

Stimulus-QRS 61 ms

Stimulus-QRS 108 ms

CHAPTER 53

Epicardial mapping and ablation of nonischemic ventricular tachycardia

James David Allred, MD *Harish Doppalapudi,* MD *&*
G. Neal Kay, MD

Clinical vignette

A 42-year-old male with nonischemic dilated cardiomyopathy and relatively well-preserved left ventricular function (left ventricular ejection fraction [LVEF] 0.45) presented with incessant ventricular tachycardia (VT). He was treated unsuccessfully with amiodarone and continued to receive multiple shocks from his implantable cardioverter defibrillator (ICD). Extensive activation mapping was precluded by hemodynamic collapse during VT. The patient was referred for cardiac transplantation due to refractory VT. However, because his primary problem was refractory arrhythmias rather than congestive heart failure, VT ablation was chosen as the more reasonable strategy.

Electrophysiology study and ablation

The patient has an idiopathic dilated cardiomyopathy and incessant VT resulting in recurrent ICD shocks despite amiodarone. His LVEF was well preserved, and so cardiac transplantation was not indicated. The QS deflection in the inferior leads of the surface ECG suggests an epicardial VT circuit (Figure 53.1). Because VT was poorly tolerated hemodynamically, an electroanatomical activation

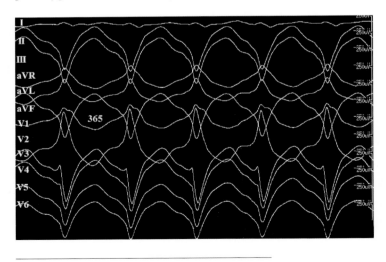

Figure 53.1 The 12-lead ECG during VT demonstrated a very wide QRS complex with right bundle branch block and right superior axis morphology. The cycle length of VT is 365 ms. The QS pattern in the inferior ECG leads is suggestive of an epicardial location of the VT circuit.

Electroanatomical Mapping, 1st edition. Edited by
A. Al-Ahmad, D. Callans, H. Hsia and A. Natale.
© 2008 Blackwell Publishing, ISBN: 9781405157025.

map was not possible. Therefore, endocardial voltage mapping was performed, which demonstrated no regions of low voltage (Figure 53.2). At the site of earliest endocardial activation there was a site where pacing closely matched the surface QRS, although the postpacing interval exceeded the VT cycle length by 20 ms and there was a short stimulus-to-QRS interval (Figure 53.3). Epicardial voltage mapping demonstrated a region of low voltage at the apex of the left ventricle (Figure 53.4). The electrograms on the epicardium demonstrated mid-diastolic potentials and the application of RF current at this site terminated VT and rendered it noninducible (Figures 53.5 and 53.6). This patient has been free of recurrent VT for over a year and has no evidence of congestive heart failure.

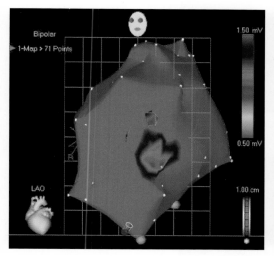

Figure 53.2 Endocardial voltage map of the left ventricle recorded during sinus rhythm demonstrates no endocardial scar.

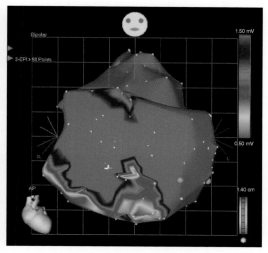

Figure 53.4 Epicardial voltage map of the left and right ventricles demonstrates a relatively small area of low voltage at the apex of the left and right ventricles.

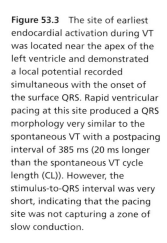

Figure 53.3 The site of earliest endocardial activation during VT was located near the apex of the left ventricle and demonstrated a local potential recorded simultaneous with the onset of the surface QRS. Rapid ventricular pacing at this site produced a QRS morphology very similar to the spontaneous VT with a postpacing interval of 385 ms (20 ms longer than the spontaneous VT cycle length (CL)). However, the stimulus-to-QRS interval was very short, indicating that the pacing site was not capturing a zone of slow conduction.

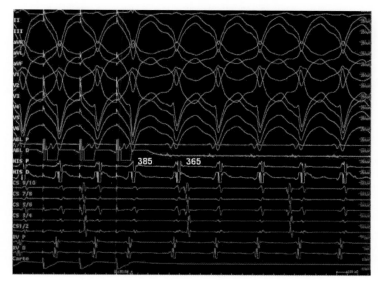

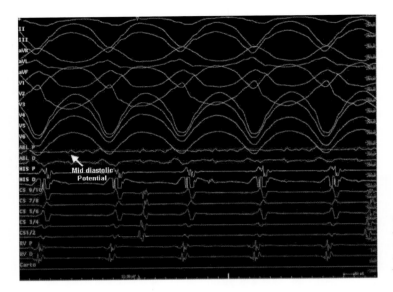

Figure 53.5   Epicardial mapping during VT demonstrated a site recording low-amplitude, mid-diastolic potentials at the apex of the left ventricle.

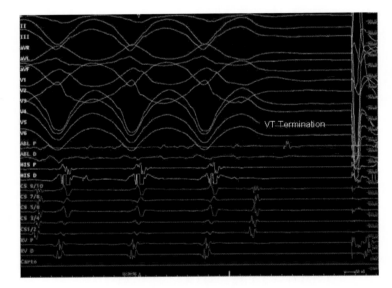

Figure 53.6   Termination of VT with RF applied to the epicardial surface of the left ventricle (same site as in Figure 53.5).

CHAPTER 54

Double-outlet right ventricle ventricular tachycardia

James David Allred, MD *Takumi Yamada,* MD, PhD
Harish Doppalapudi, MD *Yung R. Lau,* MD *& G. Neal Kay,* MD

Clinical vignette

A 12-year-old boy with a history of surgically repaired double-outlet right ventricle (DORV) with transposition of the great vessels (Taussig-Bing) and coarctation of the aorta presented with symptomatic ventricular tachycardia (VT) (Figure 54.1). The patient developed sustained rapid palpitations requiring electrical cardioversion. He was subsequently referred for catheter ablation of VT. Surgical repair included closure of a ventricular septal defect (VSD) to tunnel flow from the left ventricle to the aorta via the VSD and from the right ventricle to the pulmonary artery via the VSD (Kawashimi operation) and resection of the coarctation. Following surgical repair, the right ventricle ejects into the pulmonary artery and the left ventricle ejects into the aorta (Figures 54.2 and 54.3).

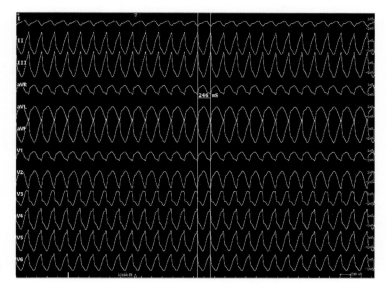

Figure 54.1 The 12-lead ECG during clinical VT demonstrates a left bundle branch block QRS morphology with right inferior axis at a cycle length of 246 ms.

Electroanatomical Mapping, 1st edition. Edited by
A. Al-Ahmad, D. Callans, H. Hsia and A. Natale.
© 2008 Blackwell Publishing, ISBN: 9781405157025.

(a)
(b)

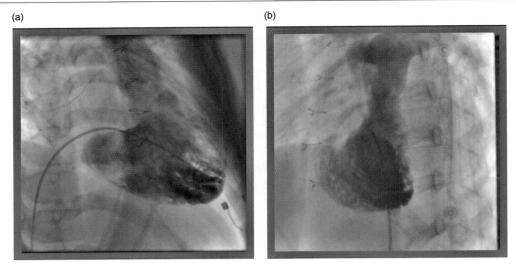

Figure 54.2 Right ventricular angiography was performed during the electrophysiology study. In the right (a) and left (b) anterior oblique projections, the pulmonary artery arises in a vertical and leftward location with a trans-annular patch and no functional valve. The aorta and pulmonary arteries have an unusual, side-by-side orientation.

(a)
(b)

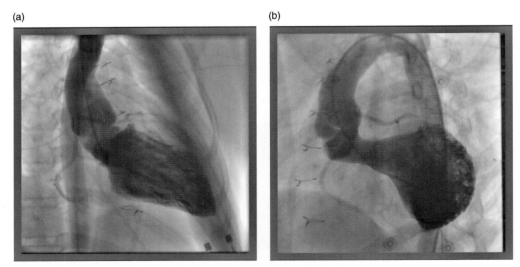

Figure 54.3 Left ventricular angiography was performed during the electrophysiology study. In the right (a) and left (b) anterior oblique projections, the aorta arises in a vertical and rightward location with a long subaortic tunnel created by the VSD closure patch. Note the anomalous origin of the left circumflex coronary artery that originates from the right coronary cusp of the aorta.

Electrophysiology study and ablation

Pacing from the anterior RV outflow tract just below the trans-annular patch reproduced an excellent pace-map (Figures 54.4 and 54.5) but VT remained inducible following RF ablation at this site. Electroanatomic mapping of the RV was performed during VT, and it revealed a centrifugal activation from the outflow tract septum where the voltage of the local ventricular electrogram was greater than 1.5 mV (Figures 54.6 and 54.7). Electroanatomic mapping of the left ventricle (LV) during the VT demonstrated centrifugal activation from the outflow tract septum (Figure 54.6). An RF application was delivered at that site in the same manner as in the RV with an interruption of the VT (Figure 54.4). During more than 6 months of

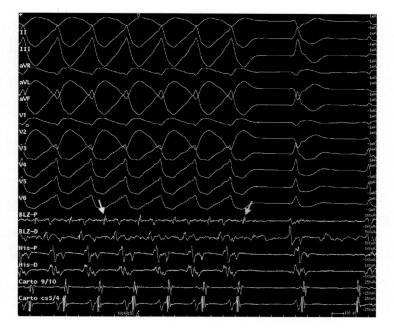

Figure 54.4 Activation mapping in the LV outflow tract demonstrates mid-diastolic activation (white arrow). The application of RF current at this site eliminated VT, though the last QRS complex is followed by the same mid-diastolic potential (yellow arrow).

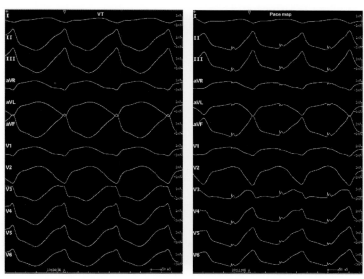

Figure 54.5 Pace-mapping from the RV outflow tract produces a close match to the clinical VT. However, catheter ablation at this site did not eliminate VT.

follow-up, the patient has been free of any ventricular arrhythmic episodes without any antiarrhythmic drugs. In this case, the VT had a focal mechanism that originated from the left ventricular septum after the complete surgical repair of the DORV. As pace-mapping in the RV was demonstrated, the preferential breakout site was considered to be located in the RV outflow tract. Therefore, the surface electrocardiogram exhibited a left bundle branch block pattern. The successful ablation site in the LV outflow tract was located in the low-voltage area, whereas the presumed preferential breakout site in the RV was located in the normal-voltage area. These findings could explain the preferential conduction from the left-side origin to the right-side breakout site. In this case, the activity of the VT origin was still observed at the successful ablation site immediately after the termination of the VT. These findings suggested that the termination of the VT might have been achieved by the isolation of the VT origin.

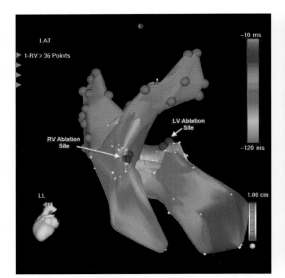

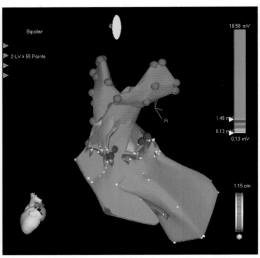

Figure 54.6   Electroanatomic mapping of the right (RV) and left (LV) ventricles and great vessels was performed using a CARTO™ mapping system during VT. Note that early activation occurs in the interventricular septal region of both the right and left ventricles.

Figure 54.7   Voltage mapping of the right and left ventricles demonstrates normal voltage without scar in the body of both ventricles. There is evidence of postoperative scarring in a small portion of the left ventricular outflow tract.

CHAPTER 55

Voltage mapping of the right ventricle in arrythmogenic right ventricular dysplasia

Kevin Makati, MD *& N. A. Mark Estes III,* MD

Clinical vignette

A 44-year-old gentleman presented after an ischemic evaluation for palpitations due to premature ventricular complexes (PVCs). A two-dimensional echocardiogram revealed the incidental finding of right ventricular enlargement. An electrocardiogram showed the presence of an epsilon waves in leads V_1–V_3 (Figure 55.1). An abnormal signal-averaged electrocardiogram (SAECG) suggested the diagnosis of arrhythmogenic right ventricular dysplasia (ARVD). The patient was taken to the electrophysiology laboratory, and a voltage map of

the right ventricle was constructed that may support the diagnosis of arrythmogenic right ventricular dysplasia.

Electrophysiology study

Electroanatomical mapping of the right ventricle revealed multiple areas of low voltage consistent with scar due to ARVD (Figure 55.2). Prior studies have suggested voltages less than 1.5 mV to be abnormal, and local electrograms within dysplastic myocardium have also been noted to be prolonged when compared with normal myocardium.

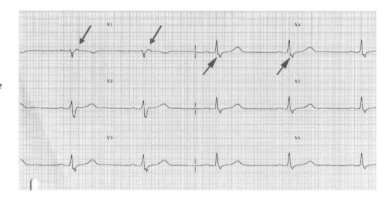

Figure 55.1 Electrocardiogram showing Epsilon waves (arrows) in the anterior (V1) and lateral (V4) precordial leads. Epsilon waves are a major diagnostic criterion and represent delayed activation of the right ventricle. It is often accompanied by a prolonged QRS interval with an incomplete or complete right bundle branch block. Although not present in these tracings, T-wave inversion is a minor criterion for the diagnosis of ARVD.

Electroanatomical Mapping, 1st edition. Edited by
A. Al-Ahmad, D. Callans, H. Hsia and A. Natale.
© 2008 Blackwell Publishing, ISBN: 9781405157025.

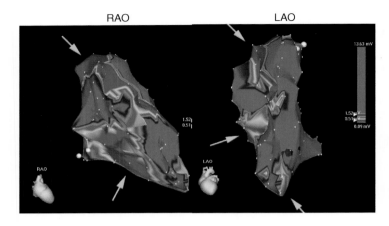

Figure 55.2 Voltage maps of the right ventricle in ARVD – right anterior oblique (RAO) projection. The voltage map shows three areas of relatively low voltage, suggesting fibrofatty replacement of myocardium (arrows): inferior, inferoapical, and infundibulum.

Electroanatomical mapping in this patient confirmed the diagnosis of ARVD with the characteristic area of scar involvement: basal perivalvular, around the right ventricular outflow tract, and on the RV free lateral wall. Voltage mapping of the right ventricle has been determined to be a useful approach in distinguishing right ventricular outflow tachycardia from ARVD as well as an adjunct to other clinical and imaging parameters.

CHAPTER 56

Ventricular tachycardia related to arrhythmogenic right ventricular dysplasia

Luis C. Sáenz, MD, *Miguel A. Vacca,* MD, MSc, *&*
Andrea Natale, MD

Clinical vignette

The patient is a 39-year-old man with recurrent tachycardia for 2 years that occurs at rest or during exercise presents with near syncope. He has no significant past medical history or familial history of sudden cardiac death. The EKG during sinus rhythm showed an incomplete right block branch and inversion of the T wave in the precordial leads (Figure 56.1a). He had previous hospitalizations because of the recurrence of the symptoms and an EKG with sustained ventricular tachycardia (VT) was obtained (Figure 56.1b). In addition to the presence of left bundle branch block VT, a diagnosis of arrhythmogenic right ventricular dysplasia (ARVD) was confirmed by RV dilatation and fat infiltration demonstrated on cardiac MRI (Figure 56.2). The patient was initially on sotalol and subsequently on amiodarone, but because of recurrent VT, he underwent a VT ablation.

Electrophysiology study and ablation

The patient was brought to the electrophysiology laboratory where a right venriculogram was

Electroanatomical Mapping, 1st edition. Edited by
A. Al-Ahmad, D. Callans, H. Hsia and A. Natale.
© 2008 Blackwell Publishing, ISBN: 9781405157025.

obtained (Figure 56.3). This confirmed the areas of abnormality seen by MRI. A CARTO™ voltage map was then generated in sinus rhythm, demonstrating an area of scar in the inferior wall of the right ventricle (Figure 56.4). VT with left bundle branch morphology and left superior axis was induced with programmed stimulation, suggesting the presence of circuit with exit from the lateral aspect of the RV inferior wall (Figure 56.5). This VT spontaneously changed to another VT that produced hypotension and was terminated by overdrive pacing. Another VT with a left bundle branch morphology and superior axis suggesting origin from a more septal aspect of the RV inferior wall (Figure 56.5) was also induced. Remarkably, the spontaneous VT could not be induced by the stimulation protocol. Mapping during VT was initially attempted. However, the frequent changing between the induced VTs and the hypotension induced by the fastest VT did prevent activation mapping. A substrate ablation strategy was performed based on the likely VT exit sites and the sinus rhythm voltage map. Electrograms recorded near the tricuspid annulus during sinus rhythm were fractionated, and near the lateral, basal region of the scar, late potentials were recorded (Figure 56.6).

Pace-mapping was performed from the borders of the inferior scar looking for the places with the best reproduction of the EKG morphology of the induced and clinical VTs (Figure 56.7).

(a)

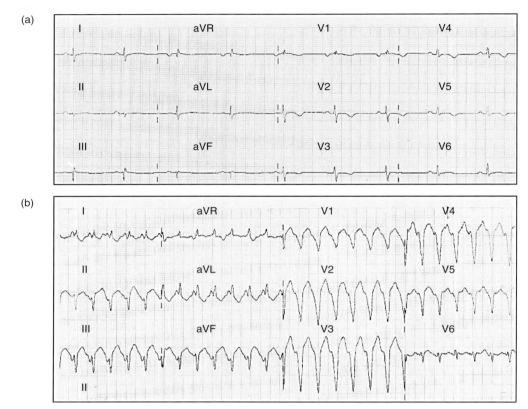

(b)

Figure 56.1 (a) EKG during sinus rhythm showing incomplete right block branch and inversion of the T wave in the precordial leads. (b) Spontaneous and recurrent VT with left bundle branch morphology and superior axis suggesting origin from the RV inferior wall.

(a)

(b)

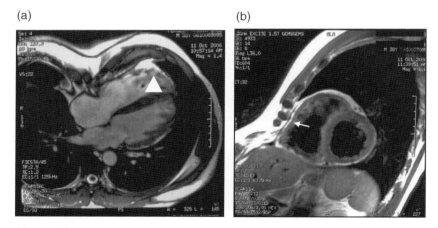

Figure 56.2 (a) MRI of this patient done before the VT ablation. Note the thinning of the right ventricle free wall (white head arrow). (b) Short axis view showing fatty infiltration of the RV (arrow) suggesting ARVD. No left ventricular abnormalities were reported.

Ablation lines were designed over the borders of the scar, crossing through the best pace-mapping points and connecting the tricuspid valve to abolish conduction over this zone (Figure 56.8). RV stimulation protocol after the ablation lines were completed and did not induce any arrhythmia. Of note, the left ventricular voltage map was completely normal (Figure 56.9).

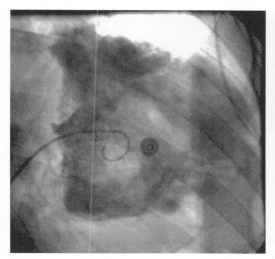

Figure 56.3   A right ventricular angiogram was done before the CARTO™ map during the VT ablation of the patient. The right anterior oblique (RAO) view shows sacculations at the RV inferior wall and the anterior aspect of RV outflow tract (RVOT) suggesting ARVD.

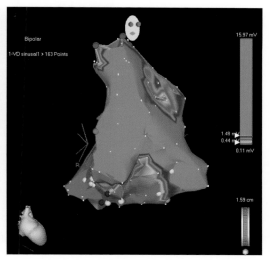

Figure 56.4   Sinus rhythm CARTO™ voltage map of the RV from the RAO view showing an inferior wall and infundibular RVOT voltage abnormalities.

(a)   (b)   (c)

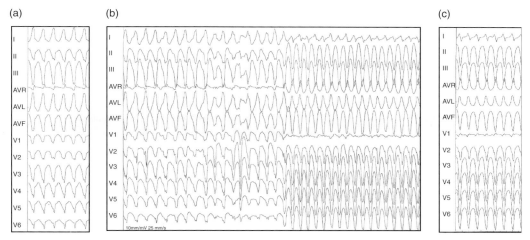

Figure 56.5   (a) VT with left bundle branch morphology and left superior axis induced, suggesting the presence of circuit with exit from the lateral aspect of the RV inferior wall. (b) This VT spontaneously changed to another VT producing hypotension requiring pace termination. (c) VT showed left bundle branch morphology and superior axis suggesting origin from a more septal aspect of the RV inferior wall.

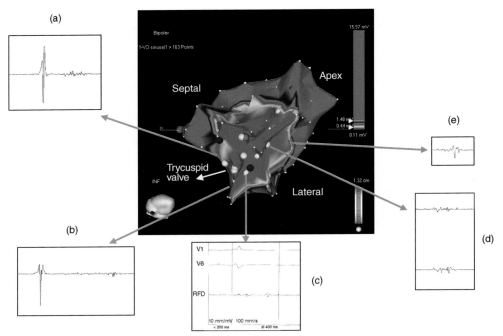

Figure 56.6 Sinus rhythm CARTO™ voltage map of the RV from the inferior view showing a scar that compromise the basal and middle segments of the inferior RV and extends to the lateral aspect. (a and b) Low amplitude and fractionated electrograms. (b) A late potential with very low amplitude and fractionated local electrical activity. These electrograms suggested a channel of abnormal tissue with very slow conduction between the inferior dense scar and the tricuspid valve (natural boundary). (c) Over the lateral aspect of the inferior scar and approximately 6 mm from the tricuspid valve site, a late potential (QRS-end of the electrogram (EGM) of 400 ms) was recorded. (d) Most of the abnormal electrograms inside the scar were recorded over the lateral aspect. (e) The recorded electrogram from the border of the scar.

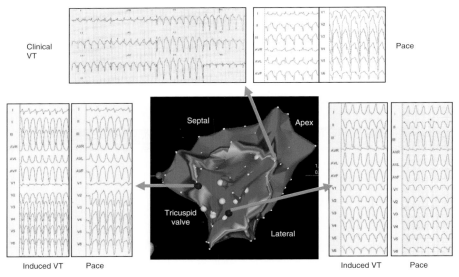

Figure 56.7 Pace-mapping was performed from the borders of the inferior scar looking for the places with the best reproduction of the EKG morphology of the induced and clinical VTs. The EKG morphology of the clinical VT (but not induced in the study) was best reproduced by the pace from the apical aspect of the scar (green dot). The EKG morphology of the induced VTs was best reproduced from the zones tagged as purple points. The more lateral best pace-mapping zone coincided with the place were the latest potential was recorded (see Figure 56.6).

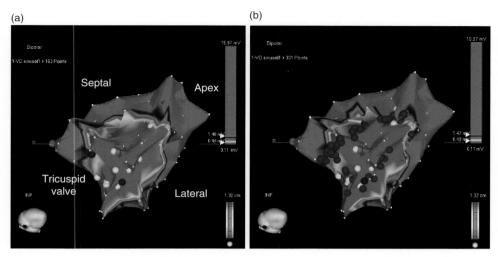

Figure 56.8   (a) Sinus rhythm CARTO™ voltage map of the RV from the inferior view showing the inferior wall scar with the pink, green, and purple dots representing the low-voltage/fractionated electrograms and the best pace-map matches of the clinical and induced VTs, respectively. (b) The linear lesions created based on the location of the presumed VT exit sites and the anatomic barrier of the tricuspid valve annulus.

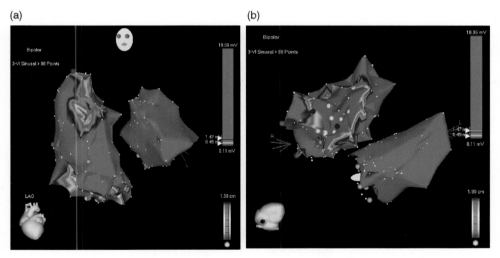

Figure 56.9   (a) Sinus rhythm CARTO™ voltage map of the RV and LV from a left anterior oblique (LAO) view. (b) Same map from an inferior view. Endocardial mapping of the LV did not reveal any abnormalities.

CHAPTER 57

Electroanatomic mapping for scar-mediated right ventricular tachycardia

Linda Huffer, MD *& William Stevenson,* MD

Clinical vignette

The patient is a 49-year-old male with a history of arrhythmogenic right ventricular dysplasia/cardiomyopathy (ARVD/C) who presented with recurrent ventricular tachycardia (VT) refractory to antiarrhythmic therapy (Figure 57.1). He initially presented at age 31 with exertional palpitations associated with sustained monomorphic VT. He was subsequently diagnosed with ARVD/C and started on medical therapy including a beta-blocker

and quinidine. He experienced recurrent VT and underwent dual-chamber implantable defibrillator implantation. Sotalol was initiated, which resulted in arrhythmia suppression for several years. He subsequently experienced recurrent VT. VT ablation was performed, which resulted in reduction in arrhythmic events for approximately 1 year. Amiodarone was then initiated, which resulted in only transient arrhythmia suppression. He was then referred for repeat electrophysiology testing and ablation. Amiodarone was discontinued, and

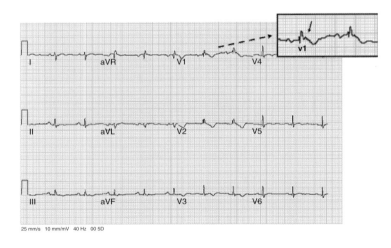

Figure 57.1 Sinus rhythm, 12-lead electrogram. The admission of 12-lead electrocardiogram demonstrates sinus rhythm with left atrial enlargement, first-degree AV block, QRS prolongation in V1 and V2 consistent with right ventricular conduction delay, T-wave inversions in V1–V4, and an epsilon wave in V1. These findings are consistent with a diagnosis of ARVD/C. The inset is an enlargement of V1 with the arrow pointing to a late systolic deflection consistent with an epsilon wave.

Electroanatomical Mapping, 1st edition. Edited by A. Al-Ahmad, D. Callans, H. Hsia and A. Natale. © 2008 Blackwell Publishing, ISBN: 9781405157025.

mexilitine was started approximately 2 months prior to elective admission. Mexilitine was held for 48 h prior to study. Incessant, hemodynamically stable, monomorphic VT (Figure 57.2) occurred during telemetry monitoring. The patient was then transferred to the electrophysiology laboratory.

An echocardiogram was obtained the day prior to electrophysiology testing, which demonstrated a left ventricular ejection fraction of 55%, moderate right atrial enlargement, moderate right ventricular enlargement, and moderately to severely reduced right ventricular function.

Electrophysiology study and ablation

The patient presented in incessant VT with a morphology and cycle length (CL) consistent with the patient's clinical tachycardia (Figure 57.3).

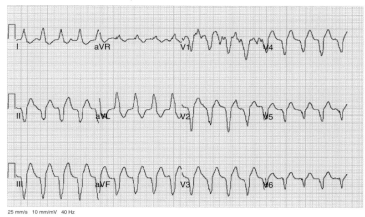

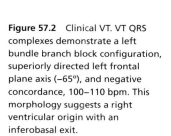

Figure 57.2 Clinical VT. VT QRS complexes demonstrate a left bundle branch block configuration, superiorly directed left frontal plane axis (−65°), and negative concordance, 100–110 bpm. This morphology suggests a right ventricular origin with an inferobasal exit.

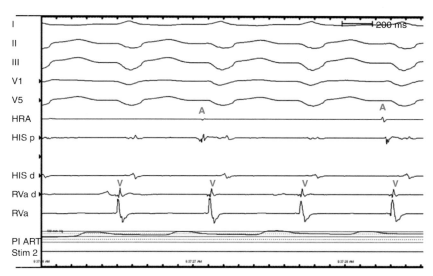

Figure 57.3 Clinical VT, intracardiac electrograms. From the top are surface electrograms leads I, II, III, V1, and V5, bipolar intracardiac electrograms recorded from the His catheter (proximal, distal), and RV apex, and the femoral arterial pressure waveform. Incessant VT with a CL of 595 ms was present upon arrival to the electrophysiology laboratory. Intracardiac electrograms demonstrate VA dissociation (2:1) consistent with a diagnosis of VT. The surface electrogram morphology was consistent with the patient's clinical tachycardia (see Figure 57.2). Note the stable femoral arterial pressure of 100/50 mmHg, which allowed for entrainment and activation mapping.

VT terminated with mechanical trauma at a site, which demonstrated split mid-diastolic potentials in both tachycardia and sinus rhythm. Sinus rhythm intervals were notable for a mildly prolonged PR interval (202 ms) and AH interval (126 ms), QRS prolongation in V1 and V2 consistent with right ventricular conduction delay, and a normal HV interval (54 ms). The clinical VT was then easily re-induced with programmed ventricular stimulation delivered from the right ventricular apex. During activation and entrainment mapping, the clinical VT repeatedly terminated and was easily re-induced.

A right ventricular electroanatomic map was then obtained in sinus rhythm using the CARTO™ system and a saline irrigated mapping and ablation catheter (Thermocool; Biosense Webster, Inc.). VT substrate was delineated by pace-mapping and annotating sites of fractionation, delay with pacing, late systolic potentials, and scar (Figures 57.4 and 57.5). Unipolar pacing at 10 mA/2 ms was utilized for pace-mapping and determination of electrically unexcitable scar (EUS). An area of low-amplitude scar with bordering EUS was present adjacent to the tricuspid valve annulus along the inferior wall of the RV. The tachycardia was stable, regular, and initially sustained allowing entrainment to be assessed from selected sites as the electroanatomic map was created. Central isthmus sites were identified. Further attempts at mapping and entrainment repeatedly resulted in VT termination or mechanical termination (Figures 57.6–57.8). Radiofrequency ablation was then applied in sinus rhythm at sites with fractionated, low-voltage late systolic potentials in the VT isthmus (Figure 57.9). The ablation lesions incorporated the central isthmus, mechanical termination, and termination by pacing sites. Repeated lesions were applied until this region was rendered electrically unexcitable (Figure 57.10). Ventricular burst pacing and programmed extrastimulation were then repeated with up to triple extrastimuli at two CLs from two sites during isoproterenol infusion. Only brief (7 s) runs of nonsustained VT with a different morphology compared with the spontaneous VT were inducible at completion of the case.

The patient remained arrhythmia free throughout the remainder of his hospital stay and was discharged on nadolol 20 mg once a day.

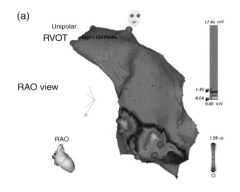

(a)

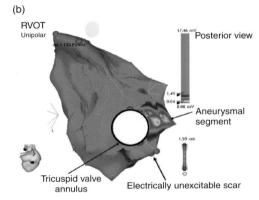

(b)

Figure 57.4 Electroanatomic map, right anterior oblique (RAO) view (a) and posterior view (b). The voltage map was constructed during sinus rhythm. Areas of EGM voltage <0.04 mV are in red. Areas of normal EGM voltage of >1.5 mV are in purple. The right ventricle was enlarged with a focal basolateral aneurysmal segment. A large region of low voltage is evident in the inferior wall and basolateral right ventricle adjacent to the tricuspid valve annulus consistent with scar. Scar secondary to fibrofatty replacement in these regions is characteristic of ARVD/C. The gray region adjacent to the septal aspect of the tricuspid valve annulus is most likely artifactual. Similarly, the EUS in the RV outflow tract (RVOT) is likely superior to the pulmonic valve.

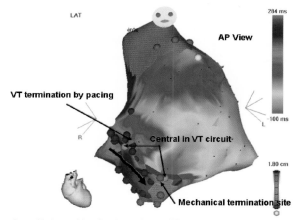

Central isthmus: blue; fractionated: pink; VT termination by pacing; aqua: mechanical termination site: red; ablation lesions: dark red; EUS: gray

Figure 57.5 VT activation map. Activation proceeds from red, to yellow, to green, to blue, to purple as the wave front proceeds superiorly from the inferior right ventricle and back through the VT isthmus in the basolateral low-voltage region. Adjacent to the mechanical termination site, earliest activation meets latest activation, characteristic of a reentry circuit. The complete circuit was not defined. Note the activation time color coded from −100 ms to 284 ms sum to 384 ms, approximately 64% of the VT CL. Successful ablation, however, was achieved. The entire reentry circuit does not need to be delineated with this approach when desirable ablation targets are identified using entrainment and substrate mapping. In addition, portions of the reentry circuit may be epicardial or intramural and not identifiable with endocardial mapping. Central isthmus, mechanical termination, and VT termination with pacing sites identified during entrainment mapping are annotated. Ablation sites are marked with dark red circles.

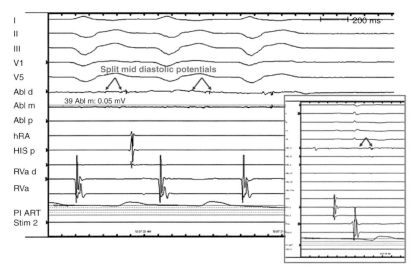

Figure 57.6 Mid-diastolic potentials at a site of VT termination with mechanical trauma. From the top are surface electrograms leads I, II, III, V1, and V5, bipolar intracardiac electrograms recorded from the ablation catheter (distal, mid, proximal), His catheter (proximal, distal), and RV apex, and the femoral arterial pressure waveform. Low-voltage (<0.05 mV) split mid-diastolic potentials were present in VT at a site where mechanical trauma terminated tachycardia without a premature ventricular contraction. Sinus rhythm at the same site, as shown in the inset, demonstrates identical late systolic split potentials. These potentials are generated by depolarization through isolated muscle fibers in scar. They are often present in a narrow isthmus in the reentry circuit at sites associated with successful ablation.

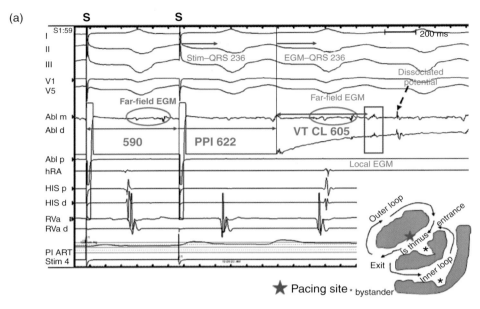

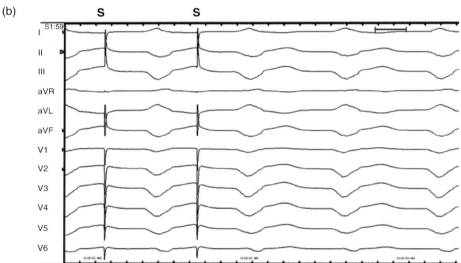

Figure 57.7   (a and b) Entrainment from a central isthmus figure. Tracings are as in Figure 57.6. The last two stimuli (S) of a train at a cycle length (CL) of 236 ms are shown followed by continuation of VT at 605 ms. The stimuli entrain VT without altering the QRS complex, consistent with entrainment with concealed fusion (ECF). The postpacing interval (PPI) (622 ms) is approximately equal to the VT CL (PPI-VT CL <30 ms), consistent with a reentry circuit site. During entrainment, the interval from the stimulus–QRS onset is 236 ms. This interval is equal to the EGM–QRS interval and is 39% of the VT tachycardia CL (TCL). These findings are consistent with entrainment from a central isthmus site. The local (blue box) and far-field (red circle) electrograms (EGMs) are labeled (a). A dissociated potential, which may be from an adjacent bystander, is seen upon termination of pacing. The 12-lead surface EKG demonstrating ECF is shown in (b).

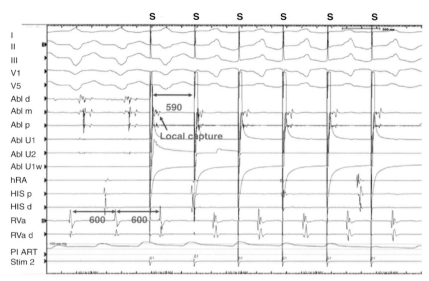

Figure 57.8   VT termination by pacing. From the top are surface electrograms leads I, II, III, V1, and V5, bipolar intracardiac electrograms recorded from the ablation catheter (distal, mid, proximal), unipolar electrograms recorded from the ablation catheter (U1, U2, U1w-unfiltered), and bipolar electrograms recorded from the His catheter (proximal, distal), and RV apex, and the femoral arterial pressure waveform. Local capture after the first stimulus results in VT termination. Unintentional VT termination is a common limitation of entrainment mapping. The second pacing stimulus results in capture with a markedly different QRS complex than during VT. These findings indicate that areas of functional block or collision of wave fronts maintain block during VT, but with termination of VT the stimulated wave front takes a different path to exit from the low-voltage region. Although the site is in the VT circuit, pace-mapping produces a marked different QRS, illustrating a potentially confusing aspect of pace-mapping for scar-related VTs.

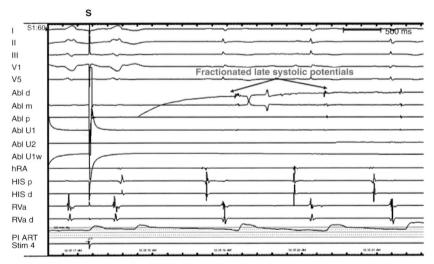

Figure 57.9   Fractionated late systolic potentials at ablation sites. Tracing are as in Figure 57.8. The last stimulus of a pacing train is shown. Pacing captures with a long S-QRS consistent with slow conduction. The electrogram is fractionated and has late potentials inscribed after the end of the QRS that are evidence of slow conduction and the likely origin of the epsilon wave in the surface ECG. RF ablation was then applied in sinus rhythm at sites with fractionated, low-voltage late systolic potentials in the VT isthmus. The ablation lesions incorporated the central isthmus, mechanical termination, and termination by pacing sites identified during entrainment mapping.

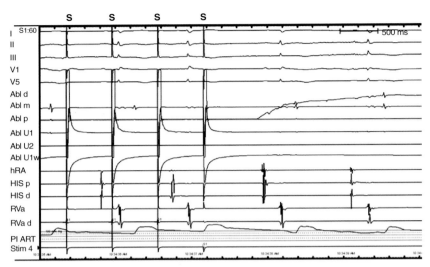

Figure 57.10   No capture after ablation. Tracing are as in Figure 57.8. Ablation was continued in the isthmus region until the area was rendered unexcitable with unipolar pacing at 10 mA/2 ms pulse width.

CHAPTER 58

Post-myocardial infarction ventricular tachycardia

John Sussman, MD

Clinical vignette

A 63-year-old male was status post-large anterior myocardial infarction with subsequent anteroapical aneurysm formation. He had a well-compensated ischemic cardiomyopathy, with left ventricular ejection fraction 20%. He developed ventricular tachycardia (VT) and underwent a successful ablation. Roughly 2 years later, he presented with frequent implantable cardioverter defibrillator (ICD) discharges for monomorphic VT, and repeat ablation was performed.

Electrophysiology study and ablation

Sinus rhythm voltage mapping revealed a large, densely infarcted, anteroapical aneurysm (Figures 58.1 and 58.2). High-density mapping showed areas of electrically unexcitable scar within the aneurysm (Figure 58.3). Programmed stimulation induced a VT with an intracardiac real-time ICD electrogram morphology identical to that recorded during arrhythmia events from the stored ICD data. Activation mapping during VT showed earliest activation just inferolateral to the channel between the areas of unexcitable scar (Figure 58.4). Entrainment mapping confirmed that the isthmus of the VT circuit ran from anterior to inferior through the channel between these areas of scar,

and ablation in this isthmus successfully terminated the tachycardia.

Programmed stimulation then induced a second VT. The high-density mapping showed additional area of electrically unexcitable scar and a channel of less densely scarred myocardium between that region and the region of unexcitable scar, which had formed the medial boundary of the isthmus of the first VT circuit (Figure 58.5). Activation mapping suggested that the tachycardia was

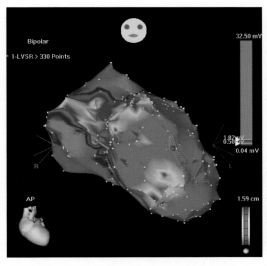

Figure 58.1 Anteroposterior (AP) view of left ventricular voltage map showed a large anteroapical aneurysm. Purple colored areas represent normal endocardium (amplitude ≥1.8 mV) with dense scar depicted as red (amplitude <0.5 mV). The gray area represents electrically unexcitable area. The border zone (amplitude 0.5–1.8 mV) is defined as areas with the intermediate color gradient.

Electroanatomical Mapping, 1st edition. Edited by A. Al-Ahmad, D. Callans, H. Hsia and A. Natale. © 2008 Blackwell Publishing, ISBN: 9781405157025.

emerging from the superior aspect of the channel between these areas (Figure 58.6). Entrainment mapping suggested that the isthmus ran from inferior to anterior through this channel. Ablation in this isthmus successfully terminated the tachycardia. Both tachycardias were rendered noninducible by the creation of lines of block across these isthmuses.

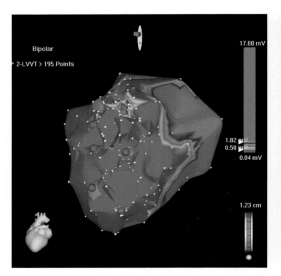

Figure 58.2 Steep left anterior oblique view of left ventricular voltage map. Gray areas denote electrically unexcitable scar.

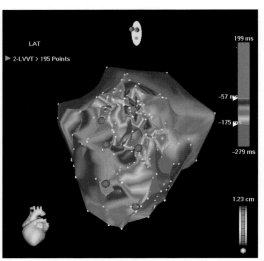

Figure 58.3 Steep left anterior oblique view of left ventricular activation map during VT. Red colored areas represent early endocardial activation with late activation depicted as blue or purple. The earliest activation was located inferolateral to the "channel" between the areas of unexcitable scar.

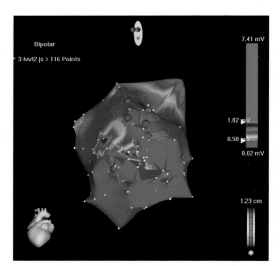

Figure 58.4 Left anterior oblique view of left ventricular voltage map. The voltage map color ranges were similar to that of Figure 58.3. Gray areas denote electrically unexcitable scar within the anteroapical aneurysm.

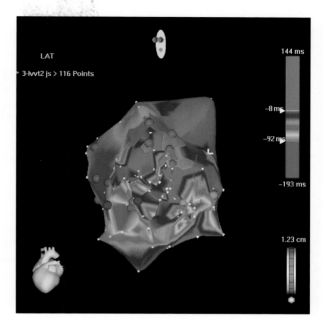

Figure 58.5   Left anterior oblique view of left ventricular activation map during second VT; gray areas denote electrically unexcitable scar. Activation map color ranges were similar to that of Figure 58.4. Activation mapping suggested that the tachycardia was emerging from the superior aspect of the channel between these areas.

CHAPTER 59

Endocardial and epicardial ventricular tachycardia ablation

Daejoon Anh, MD *Paul C. Zei,* MD *& Henry Hsia,* MD

Clinical vignette

A 54-year-old man from Nicaragua with newly diagnosed idiopathic cardiomyopathy presented with sustained ventricular tachycardia (left bundle left superior axis morphology, cycle length 440 ms), causing hemodynamic collapse requiring mechanical ventilation and inotropic support. After failed external cardioversion attempts, intravenous amiodarone and lidocaine were used to terminate the arrhythmia, although the clinical course was marked with frequent recurrences of the ventricular tachycardia (VT).

Electrophysiology study and ablation

Substrate mapping of the left ventricle in sinus rhythm did not demonstrate significant areas of scar (Figure 59.1), although areas with late potentials were found in the inferior septum. The clinical arrhythmia was inducible and endocardial mapping and radiofrequency ablation lesions were delivered, although the VT remained inducible at the end of the procedure. An implantable cardioverter defibrillator (ICD) was implanted and the patient was discharged on amiodarone.

The patient was free from VT initially, but had several recurrences 6 months after the initial procedure, requiring multiple ICD shocks. A second

electrophysiology study with epicardial substrate mapping revealed an epicardial posterior LV scar (red colored areas, Figure 59.2a and b). In addition, many areas within the scar demonstrated late potentials in sinus rhythm. The substrate map was further refined by registering points where high-output unipolar pacing failed to excite the local myocardium (Figure 59.3). Radiofrequency ablation guided by entrainment and pace-mapping adjacent to the electrically unexcitable scar led to the successful ablation of the VT, with no subsequent recurrence to date.

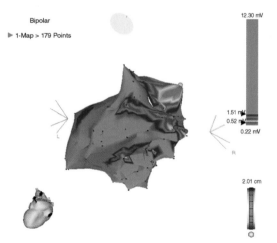

Figure 59.1 Endocardial three-dimensional CARTO™ voltage map of the left ventricle is displayed in posterior view. The purple dots (red arrow) represent sites that demonstrated late potentials in sinus rhythm. These potentials were not associated with an area of myocardial scar, consistent with relatively normal endocardium contiguous with a scarred epicardium.

Electroanatomical Mapping, 1st edition. Edited by A. Al-Ahmad, D. Callans, H. Hsia and A. Natale.
© 2008 Blackwell Publishing, ISBN: 9781405157025.

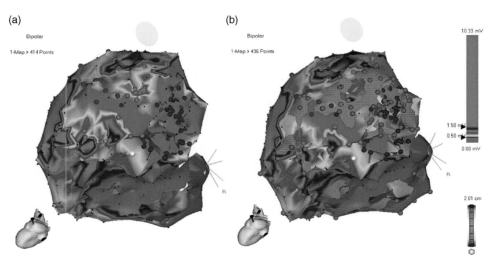

Figure 59.2   (a) CARTO™ voltage map of the left ventricular epicardial surface in posterior view. The red colored areas demonstrates large posterior scar (local electrogram amplitude less than 0.5 mV). The right ventricle (not shown) did not demonstrate any low-voltage areas. The purple dots indicate sites where late potentials were recorded in sinus rhythm. A reasonable pace-map of the VT at the inferior edge of the scar was obtained, with stimulus–QRS interval consistent with an exit site (<30% of the VT cycle length). Sites where phrenic nerve was captured with high-output unipolar pacing were marked with green dots. (b) Electrically unexcitable scar (gray dots, defined by the absence of local capture with unipolar pacing at 10 mA output) is superimposed upon the bipolar voltage map seen in Figure 59.2a. Channels of conducting tissue bounded by electrically unexcitable areas are identified, representing potential VT isthmus sites. Entrainment near the electrically unexcitable scar identified areas close to the entrance of the VT circuit (red arrow, corresponding intracardiac tracing is shown in Figure 59.3). Radiofrequency ablations (red dots) performed between the entrance and exit sites rendered the VT completely noninducible.

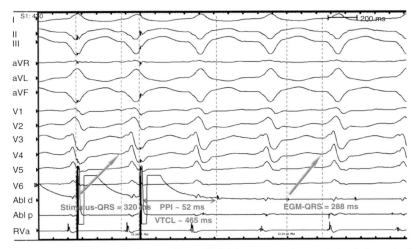

Figure 59.3   Unipolar pacing at this site (red arrow, Figure 59.2b) demonstrated concealed entrainment, stimulus–QRS interval was within 30 ms of EGM–QRS interval, with some beat-to-beat variations. The stimulus–QRS interval was >70% of the VT cycle length, consistent with an entrance site. Radiofrequency ablation at this site terminated the VT, although VT still remained inducible after this initial ablation. Ablation of areas between the entrance and the exit exhibiting local capture with high-output unipolar pacing ultimately led to noninducibility of the VT.

CHAPTER 60

Ablation of ventricular tachycardia in the setting of coronary artery disease using dynamic substrate mapping

David Callans, MD, FACC, FHRS

Clinical vignette

A 67-year-old man was referred for management of fairly well-tolerated incessant left-bundle-left-superior axis (LBLS) ventricular tachycardia (VT) with a cycle length of 380 ms. He had a history of a small remote inferior infarction and an ejection fraction of 40%. On arrival to the electrophysiology laboratory, he was in sinus rhythm, and despite incessant VT for the 3 days prior, LBLS VT could not be induced. A right-bundle-right-superior axis (RBRS) VT was easily induced.

Electrophysiology study and ablation

Using the EnSite Array, dynamic substrate mapping was employed. This method quickly outlines the boundaries of the infarct from isopotential maps in sinus rhythm and/or pacing. In Figure 60.1, the substrate, defined by late, low-voltage activation in sinus rhythm, is outlined by a gray line. Attention was directed to how activation patterns during VT interacted with the area defined as by dynamic substrate mapping. It was found that activation during VT appeared to enter and exit the substrate at relatively discrete areas, as shown in Figures 60.2 and 60.3. Interestingly, pacing at the site of entrance during VT matched the QRS morphology of the LBLS VT (the clinical, but noninducible morphology), suggesting that these VTs were "paired," related to the same substrate anatomy.

Several ablation lesions placed at the area of the exit from the substrate terminated the tachycardia and prevented inducible VT of any morphology.

Electroanatomical Mapping, 1st edition. Edited by
A. Al-Ahmad, D. Callans, H. Hsia and A. Natale.
© 2008 Blackwell Publishing, ISBN: 9781405157025.

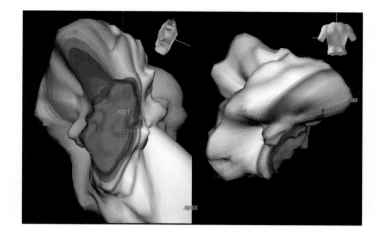

Figure 60.1 Dynamic substrate mapping (DSM) outlining an area of late activation (gray circle) suggestive of the presence of infarct-related substrate.

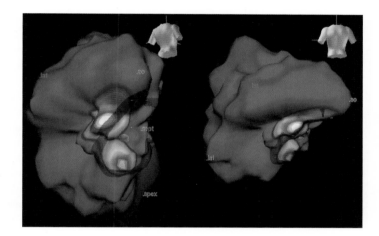

Figure 60.2 VT entrance to the substrate. Unipolar activation maps during VT using the noncontact array. Activation during VT appeared to enter and exit the "substrate" area defined by DSM at relatively discrete locations.

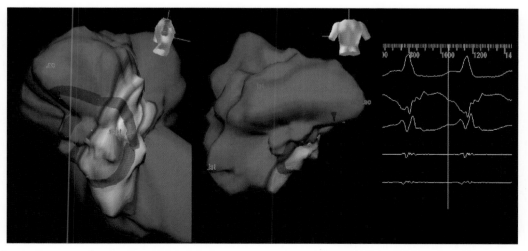

Figure 60.3 VT exit from the substrate. Unipolar activation maps during VT using the noncontact array that demonstrated the earliest activation and exit from the "substrate" area defined by DSM.

CHAPTER 61

Endocardial and epicardial mapping for ischemic ventricular tachycardia

Tamer S. Fahmy, MD, *Oussama M. Wazni,* MD, *Moataz Ali,* MD, *Robert A. Schweikert,* MD, *& Andrea Natale,* MD

Clinical vignette

The patient is a 58-year-old male who has been referred for ablation of ventricular tachycardia (VT). His history is significant for an old myocardial infarction followed by ischemic cardiomyopathy, and he underwent implantation of a biventricular defibrillator for resynchronization therapy. He suffered repeated episodes of VT, which was resistant to different antiarrhythmic medications and required repeated shocks. One year ago, an ablation procedure for his VT was attempted; however, VT episodes

recurred again and he received 15 shocks over a period of 48 h. His ECG during tachycardia had a right bundle branch block (RBBB) morphology with superior axis (Figure 61.1). His echocardiography revealed markedly dilated LV with severe impairment of contractility (EF=16%). The patient was evaluated for underlying ischemia prior to the ablation procedure. A positron emission tomography (PET) scan revealed evidence of scar in the inferior wall (12%), and hibernating myocardium in the lateral and inferolateral walls (25% of the LV). He was considered for another attempt of VT ablation.

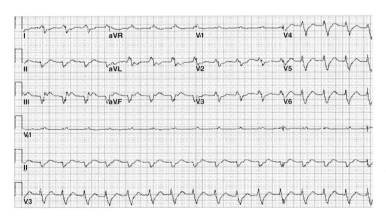

Figure 61.1 The 12-lead ECG during tachycardia having atypical RBBB morphology with superior axis. This appeared to be originating from the inferolateral wall of the LV.

Electroanatomical Mapping, 1st edition. Edited by A. Al-Ahmad, D. Callans, H. Hsia and A. Natale.
© 2008 Blackwell Publishing, ISBN: 9781405157025.

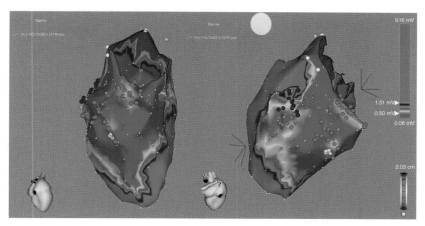

Figure 61.2   Voltage map of the LV in inferior view (left) and left posterior oblique (LPO) view (right). At the conventional scar setting (healthy myocardium >1.5 mV and scar <0.5 mV), a large scar area is seen involving the inferior, inferolateral, and a small septal area. The anterior and anterolateral walls seem healthy.

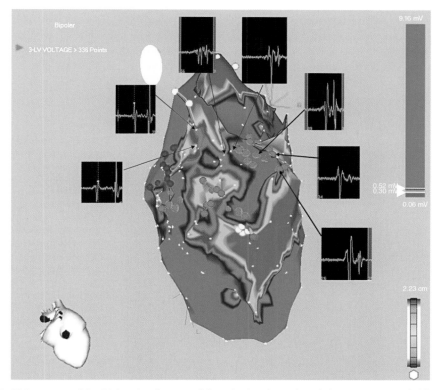

Figure 61.3   Voltage map of the LV showing the potential conducting channels and electrograms recorded from these sites. The scar settings have been changed to visualize channels (>0.5 mV "nonscar"; <0.3 mV dense scar). As shown, there is a corridor of double potentials seen during right ventricular paced rhythm. Within the scar area the double potentials are separated from each other, while within the channels they are close to each other indicating less local conduction delay within the channels. Note that the double potential at the border of the channels has a large electrogram followed by a smaller local delayed potential, whereas the recordings within the channels have larger late local electrogram components. In addition, the timing between the double potentials is also longer on the lateral wall (left) than the septal wall (right), which may reflect the wave front of activation from RV to LV during RV pacing.

Electrophysiology study and ablation

The patient underlying rhythm in the electrophysiology (EP) lab was biventricularly paced. He had easily inducible VT, with at least three different morphologies. With a retrograde aortic approach, extensive endocardial voltage mapping (475 sampled points) during paced rhythm was performed (CARTO™ system and Navistar ThermoCool catheter). This revealed basal to mid-posterior scar that extended to the posterolateral and posteroseptal regions. The remainder of the LV, particularly anteriorly, anterolaterally, and anteroseptally, demonstrated no significant scar (Figure 61.2). There were three regions of denser scar (<0.3 mV), with narrow areas between them of diseased but potentially more viable tissue (Figures 61.3 and 61.4). Pacing from these regions approximated the VT morphology at some points with long stimulus-to-QRS delay similar to that seen of the electrogram-to-QRS during VT. Having an inferior scar with multiple VT morphologies, the right ventricle was also mapped with a small inferior scar. Given the multiple induced VT morphologies as well as a prior failed attempt of ablation, a decision was made to perform epicardial mapping. Percutaneous pericardial access was obtained with a subxiphoid approach using an epidural needle. Epicardial voltage mapping was performed with about 350 sample points acquired (Figure 61.5). This demonstrated a much smaller posterior epicardial scar compared with the endocardial scar and no regions of fractionated or mid-diastolic potentials. However, the epicardial scar extended on the right side more than the endocardial RV scar. Focusing on the LV endocardial approach, lines of RF lesions were delivered, connecting the three regions of scar crossing over the more viable regions in between, and also a line from the scar up to the mitral annulus posteriorly (Figure 61.6). Post-ablation, there were no longer inducible VT with programmed ventricular stimulation with up to three extrastimuli or with ventricular burst pacing.

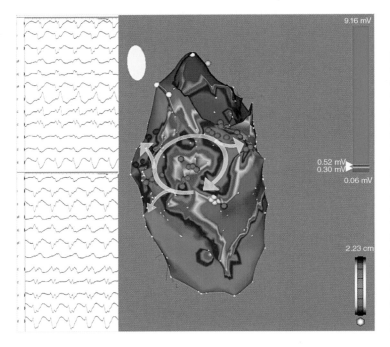

Figure 61.4 Voltage mapping of the LV. The scar settings have been changed to visualize possible channels within the scar area. Areas in red are dense scars having a voltage less than 0.3 mV, while purple areas have voltage greater than 0.5 mV. As shown there are three dense scar areas, with potential "channels" interspersed. The endocardial "channels" have voltage ranges (>0.5 mV) higher than that of the surrounding tissues (<0.3 mV). The densely scarred areas form the barriers around which the tachycardia may rotate within the less-diseased tissues. On the left, two tachycardias are shown with slightly different morphologies arising from different exits on the inferolateral border.

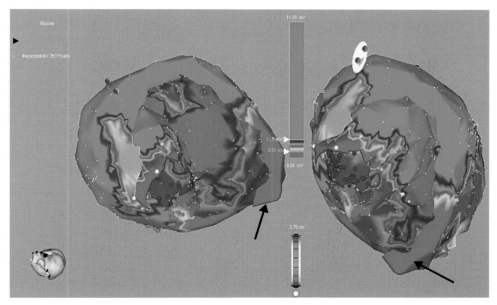

Figure 61.5   Voltage map of the endocardium and pericardium. As shown, the area of scar epicardially coincides with, although smaller than, that in the LV endocardium. There is another scar area overlying the RV (arrow).

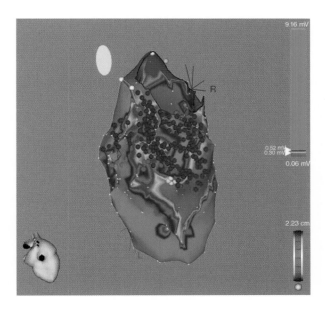

Figure 61.6   Voltage map with the same setting (0.3–0.5 mV) showing the ablation lesions created. The ablation lines were designed to connect the dense scar areas crossing over the corridor of relatively healthy tissue, as well as connecting the dense scar to the mitral valve.

CHAPTER 62

Electroanatomical mapping for ischemic ventricular tachycardia

Henry Hsia, MD

Clinical vignette

A 78-year-old man with coronary artery disease, prior myocardial infarctions and an ischemic cardiomyopathy had recurrent episodes of monomorphic ventricular tachycardia (VT) that required multiple implantable cardioverter defibrillator (ICD) shocks. He failed amiodarone and had a previous unsuccessful catheter ablation attempt.

He was treated with sotalol but presented with a sustained wide-complex tachycardia at a cycle length of 340 ms (Figure 62.1). The tachycardia was poorly tolerated and required cardioversion to restore sinus rhythm.

Noninvasive imaging stress test showed a large anterior scar without ischemia. An echocardiogram showed an ejection fraction of 35% with multiple wall motion abnormalities without apical thrombus.

LBB-Left-Inferior (LBL) VT

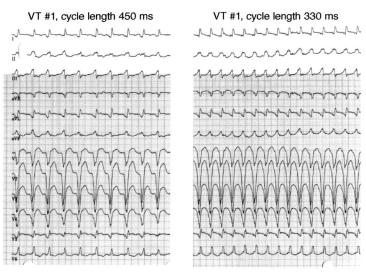

VT #1, cycle length 450 ms

VT #1, cycle length 330 ms

Figure 62.1 Left-bundle-branch-left-inferior (LBLI) VT at two different rates but were otherwise identical. Patient's presenting arrhythmia had a cycle length of 340 ms.

Electroanatomical Mapping, 1st edition. Edited by
A. Al-Ahmad, D. Callans, H. Hsia and A. Natale.
© 2008 Blackwell Publishing, ISBN: 9781405157025.

Electrophysiology study and ablation

A limited activation map was performed during VT and a detailed endocardial voltage map was constructed during sinus rhythm. Activation mapping, pace-mapping, and entrainment mapping were performed, coupled with the voltage profiles for characterization of the electroanatomic substrate (Figures 62.2–62.6). Progressively longer stimulus–QRS/electrogram–QRS intervals were tagged that extended from the circuit exit site into the dense scar toward the entrance.

VTs with identical morphologies but different rates may represent different circuits with the same exit sites, or "double reentry" with two wave fronts coexist within one circuit. Ablation lesion delivery was designed to ablate areas with higher voltage compared with surrounding tissues. VT was no longer inducible after the ablation.

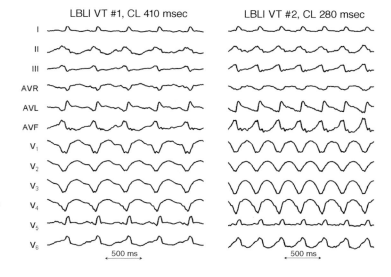

Figure 62.2   During electrophysiology study, an LBLI VT similar to patient's clinical arrhythmia was induced. Two different VT rates with cycle lengths of 410 ms and 280 ms were recorded.

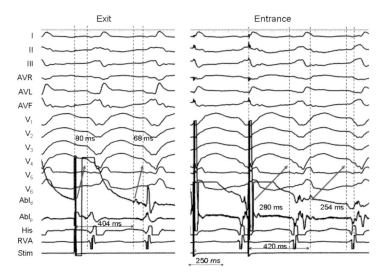

Figure 62.3   Entrainment with concealed fusion. The exit site is identified with a short stimulus–QRS interval and minimal surface fusion. The entrance site is identified with a perfect entrainment response with a long stimulus–QRS interval matches that of electrogram–QRS interval.

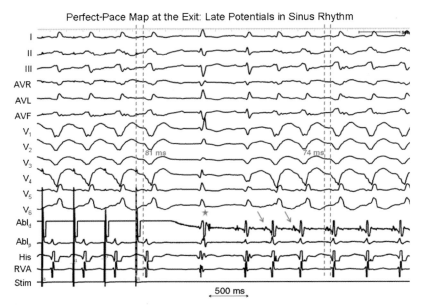

Figure 62.4 Pace-map with an exact paced QRS morphology as that of spontaneous VT. The stimulus–QRS (81 ms) approximates the electrogram–QRS (74 ms). A late potential (*) was present at this site during a single sinus beat after pacing. Of note, spontaneous VT initiation occurred after a single sinus beat with presystolic potentials that correspond to an exit site during reentrant VT. The first beat of VT is actually a fusion beat that may represent a "concealed" initiation of reentry.

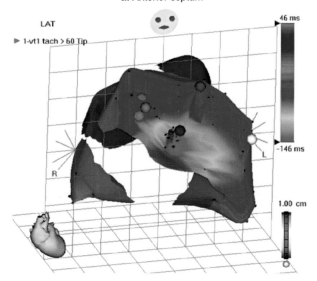

Figure 62.5 Limited activation map of the LBLI VT. The earliest endocardial activation is depicted by the red color, which was located at the anterior septum.

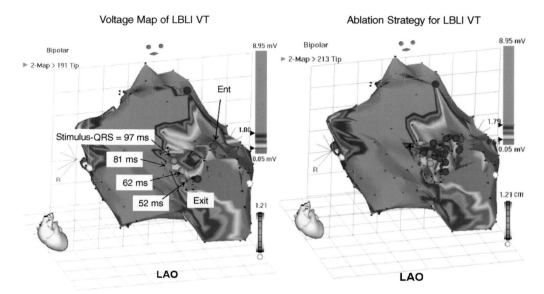

Figure 62.6   Detailed characterization of the electroanatomic substrate. Voltage map coupled with activation, entrainment, and pace-mapping define part of the VT circuit. Entrance resides deep in the dense scar whereas the exit is closer to the border zone. Ablation lesion delivery was designed to ablate areas with higher voltage compared with surrounding tissues.

CHAPTER 63

Electroanatomical mapping for scar-based reentrant ventricular tachycardia

Henry A. Chen, MD *& Henry H. Hsia,* MD

Clinical vignette

A 51-year-old male was admitted with sustained ventricular tachycardia (VT) 1 month after myocardial infarction. The patient had a large anterior wall myocardial infarction and underwent placement of a stent in the left anterior descending artery. His ejection fraction after the infarct was 25%. He had an implantable cardioverter defibrillator (ICD) implantation 1 month after his infarction. A repeat catheterization revealed no new critical coronary stenosis. Multiple antiarrhythmic agents were attempted including sotalol, amiodarone, dofetilide, lidocaine, and procainamide. The patient continued to have recurrent sustained ventricular tachycardia at a rate of approximately 170 bpm (Figure 63.1), requiring repeated ICD shocks. He was transferred to our institution for VT ablation.

Electrophysiology study and ablation

Electrode catheters were placed to the His bundle region and right ventricular apex, and mapping was performed in the left ventricle. Voltage mapping was performed to delineate areas of scar. A ventricular tachycardia with a right-bundle-right-superior axis (RBRS) morphology was easily induced. Activation, entrainment, and pace-mapping were performed to identify the components of the circuit (Figures 63.2 and 62.3). During the study, another morphology was induced (right-bundle-right-inferior axis, RBRI), of which isthmus site was also identified (Figure 63.4). Linear ablation was performed between the identified areas of exit and isthmus (Figures 63.5 and 62.6). No further VT was inducible after completion of the linear lesions through the large anterior scar.

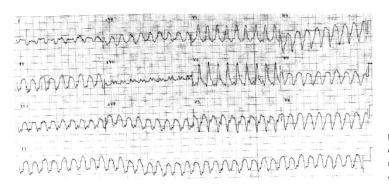

Figure 63.1 The 12-lead electrocardiogram during VT. RBRS morphology with cycle length approximately 470 ms.

Electroanatomical Mapping, 1st edition. Edited by
A. Al-Ahmad, D. Callans, H. Hsia and A. Natale.
© 2008 Blackwell Publishing, ISBN: 9781405157025.

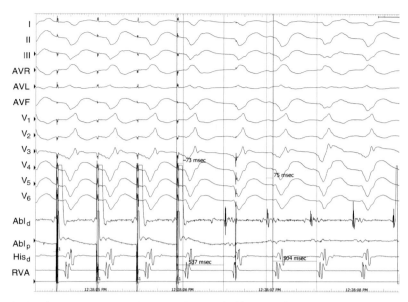

Figure 63.2   Exit site of RBRS VT. Note entrainment with concealed fusion at this site.

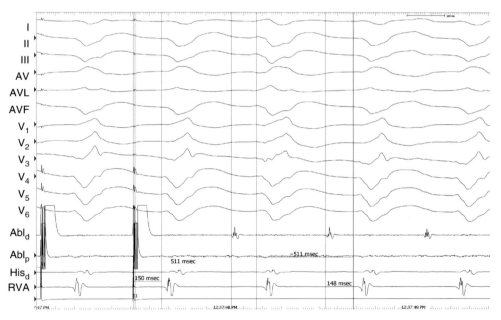

Figure 63.3   Isthmus site of RBRS VT: Entrainment with concealed fusion with an identical paced QRS morphology compared to the spontaneous VT, along with a long stimulus–QRS interval that equals to the electrogram–QRS interval of ~150 ms.

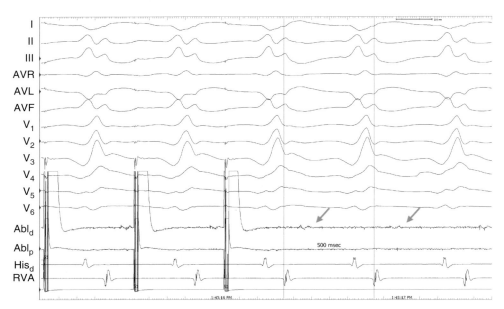

Figure 63.4 Second VT induced (RBRI morphology). Isthmus site identified with entrainment with concealed fusion with long stimulus–QRS time. Note the extremely low amplitude, fractionated signals recorded at the ablation catheter (arrow).

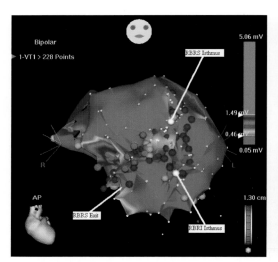

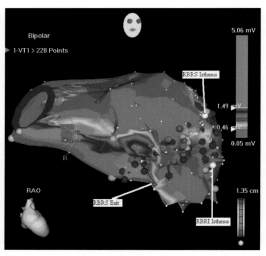

Figure 63.5 Anterior-posterior (AP) view of a LV electroanatomic voltage map showing a large area of anterior scar and the isthmus area targeted for ablation. Linear ablation lesions were delivered to connect the isthmus and the exit site for the RBRS VT, as well as connecting the RBRI VT isthmus to the RBRS isthmus sites.

Figure 63.6 Right anterior oblique (RAO) view of the LV voltage map. Lesions were delivered over scar in linear fashion from the site identified as isthmus of RBRS VT to its exit and to the site identified as RBRI isthmus.

CHAPTER 64

Electroanatomical mapping for scar-based reentrant ventricular tachycardia

Henry A. Chen, MD *& Henry H. Hsia,* MD

Clinical vignette

A 58-year-old man with a history of coronary artery disease, prior anterior myocardial infarction, and implantable cardioverter defibrillator (ICD) implantation for sustained ventricular tachycardia (VT) was admitted with ICD therapy including shock due to multiple episodes of VT (>100 episodes within 6 months). Cardiac catheterization demonstrated nonocclusive coronary disease, an anteroseptal aneurysm, and ejection fraction of 35%. The patient's clinical VT episodes were right-bundle-right-inferior (RBRI) axis morphology with a cycle length of 350–370 ms (Figure 64.1). He continued to have VT despite treatment with multiple antiarrhythmic medications including amiodarone and was referred for catheter ablation.

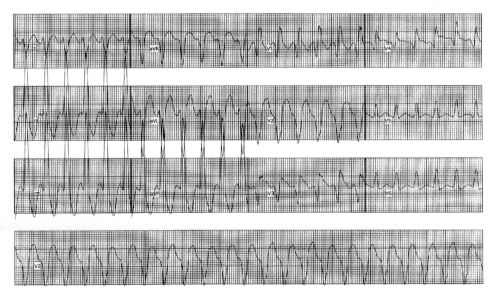

Figure 64.1 Surface ECG of spontaneous VT. RBRI-QRS axis morphology.

Electroanatomical Mapping, 1st edition. Edited by
A. Al-Ahmad, D. Callans, H. Hsia and A. Natale.
© 2008 Blackwell Publishing, ISBN: 9781405157025.

Electrophysiology study and ablation

Electrode catheters were placed in the His bundle region and right ventricular apex, and mapping was performed in the left ventricle. Sinus rhythm voltage mapping was performed to delineate areas of scar. There was a dense septal-apical aneurysm, consistent with echocardiographic findings (Figure 64.2). A RBRI axis VT was induced, which matched the clinical morphology. Activation mapping and pace-mapping were performed (Figure 64.3) and

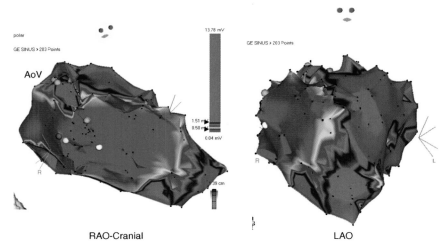

Figure 64.2 Voltage mapping constructed during sinus rhythm demonstrating a dense septal-apical aneurysm. Purple colored areas represent normal endocardium (amplitude ≥1.5 mV) with dense scar depicted as red (amplitude <0.5 mV). The border zone (amplitude 0.5–1.5 mV) is defined as areas with the intermediate color gradient.

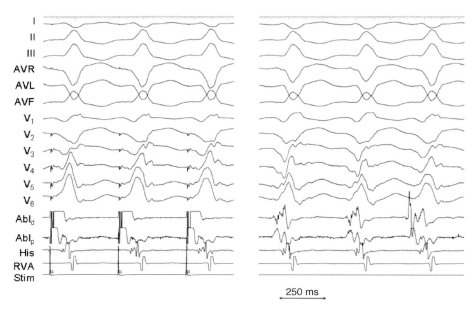

Figure 64.3 Pace-mapping (left panel) was performed at a site within a potentially conducting channel within the scar. This area was identified as an exit site by its morphological match to the clinical VT (right panel). The short stimulation-to-QRS time is consistent with an exit site rather than a site more proximal within the circuit.

identified the exit site in the "border zone" of the scar (Figure 64.4). A presumed "channel" of preferentially conducting tissue within the scar was identified by detailed voltage mapping and careful color threshold adjustment. More detailed activation and entrainment mapping were performed at sites within the potentially conducting channels to delineate other components of the circuit. VT terminated within 1.1 s of RF energy delivery, with successful ablation at the isthmus site. Linear ablation was performed between the identified areas of VT exit and the VT isthmus (Figures 64.5 and 64.6). Following ablation, the patient was no longer inducible.

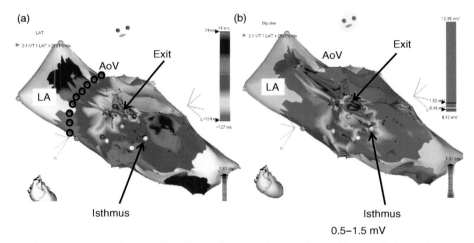

Figure 64.4   (a) Activation map during RBRI VT. The earliest activation was depicted in red with blue color representing late activation. The three-dimensional endocardial chamber construction included left atrial space and an arbitrary line was placed to outline the approximate location of the mitral valve plane. (b) LV bipolar voltage map constructed during VT. Standard color ranges were displayed with purple colored areas representing normal endocardium (≥1.5 mV) and dense scar depicted as red (<0.5 mV). Note that the VT exit site is located at the border zone (intermediate colors) with electrogram amplitudes between 0.5 mV and 1.5 mV.

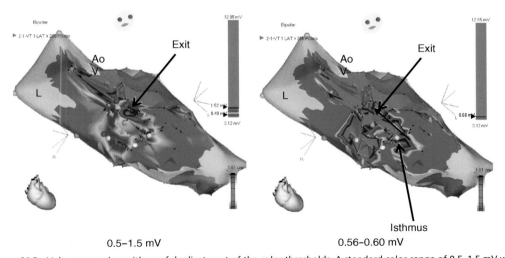

Figure 64.5   Voltage mapping with careful adjustment of the color thresholds. A standard color range of 0.5–1.5 mV was depicted on the left panel. With color range set at 0.56–0.60 mV, a potential conducting channel with higher local electrogram voltages within the "channel" (>0.60 mV) compared to the surrounding tissues (<0.56 mV) was identified. An isthmus site was located more proximal into the channel. Ablation lesions were delivered in a linear pattern between isthmus to exit area. Following ablation the patient was no longer inducible.

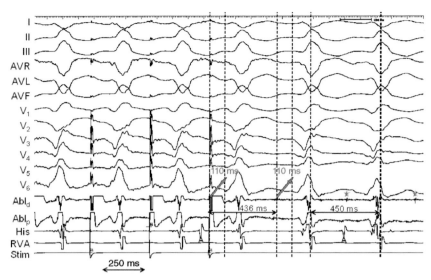

Figure 64.6 Mapping catheter positioned in septal left ventricle, deep into the "channel": entrainment with concealed fusion confirmed the isthmus site. Noticeable mid-diastolic potentials with orthodromic capture.

CHAPTER 65

Epicardial mapping and ablation of ischemic ventricular tachycardia

James David Allred, MD *Harish Doppalapudi,* MD *&*
G. Neal Kay, MD

Clinical vignette

A 59-year-old male with a prior inferior myocardial infarction was admitted for emergent ablation for incessant ventricular tachycardia (VT). The patient experienced multiple episodes of sustained VT over the previous 2 weeks. He was treated with amiodarone, mexiletine, and procainamide, and had received multiple implantable cardioverter defibrillator (ICD) shocks. Despite this, he remained in slow monomorphic VT at a rate of 120 bpm, which was below the programmed VT detection rate. Two endocardial VT ablation procedures before transfer did not influence the VT.

Electrophysiology study and ablation

The mapping and ablation strategy was to initially create a voltage map of the endocardial surface of the left ventricle to identify regions of scarred myocardium. Because there was very little evidence for endocardial scar, an epicardial voltage map was created using an irrigated-tip, electroanatomic mapping catheter (Biosense Webster Carto Thermocool). Epicardial mapping demonstrated a much more extensive region of low-voltage electrograms (Figures 65.1 and 65.2). The local electrograms in the epicardial surface showed mid-diastolic potentials with a large interval between potentials recorded from the proximal and distal electrode pairs. Transient entrainment at this site demonstrated entrainment with concealed fusion and catheter ablation at this site terminated VT and rendered all VT noninducible. There was evidence that the endocardial surface was minimally scarred with only a small region of low voltage near the mitral valve annulus. When the classic criteria for transient entrainment are fulfilled, a reentrant mechanism is proven and the goal of the ablation strategy should be to find the slowly conducting zone within the circuit. Epicardial mapping demonstrated electrograms that spanned much of diastole, suggesting that the catheter was located within a region of slow conduction (Figure 65.3). However, to prove that this slowly conducting zone was actually involved within the tachycardia circuit and not a simple bystander, the response to rapid pacing is needed (Figure 65.4). Transient entrainment was highly predictive that the ablation catheter was well positioned within the slowly conducting zone of the circuit by the criteria: (1) the postpacing interval was similar to the VT cycle length; (2) there was no change in the captured QRS morphology; (3) mid-diastolic electrograms were recorded; and (4) there was a long stimulus-to-QRS interval that was similar to the local electrogram-to-QRS interval during spontaneous VT. Epicardial ablation terminated this VT and rendered all VT noninducible (Figure 65.5). The patient has had no recurrence of VT for over a year following ablation.

Electroanatomical Mapping, 1st edition. Edited by
A. Al-Ahmad, D. Callans, H. Hsia and A. Natale.
© 2008 Blackwell Publishing, ISBN: 9781405157025.

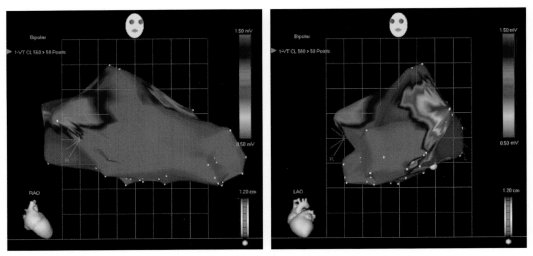

Figure 65.1   An electroanatomic voltage map in right anterior oblique (RAO) (A) and left anterior oblique (LAO) (B) views was created within the cavity of the left ventricle with a voltage range set to 0.5–1.5 mV. Note that the endocardial voltage demonstrates minimal evidence for scar that is confined to the posterior basal left ventricle near the mitral valve annulus.

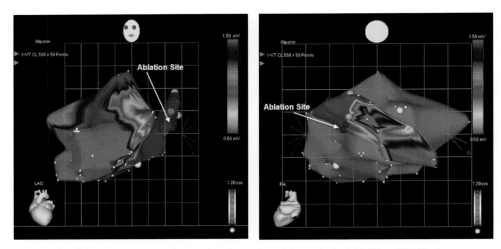

Figure 65.2   Epicardial voltage map superimposed on the endocardial map in the LAO (A) and PA (B) views demonstrating scar in the posterior basal left ventricle near the mitral annulus. Note that the region of scar on the epicardial surface is larger than on the endocardial surface. The site of catheter ablation is shown on the epicardial surface.

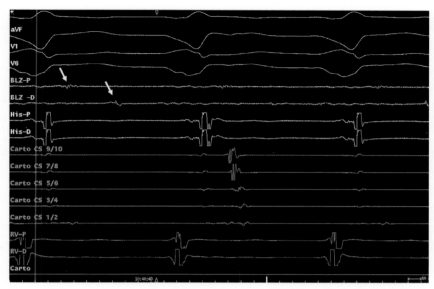

Figure 65.3 Surface electrocardiographic leads I, aVF, and V1 are shown with simultaneous bipolar electrograms recorded from the proximal (BLZ-P) and distal (BLZ-D) electrode pairs of a quadrapolar irrigated epicardial ablation catheter. Note the marked separation of diastolic potentials in the proximal and distal electrograms (arrows), suggesting that the proximal pair was recorded from the entrance point of a slowly conducting channel while the distal pair was recorded from the mid-portion of the slow conduction zone.

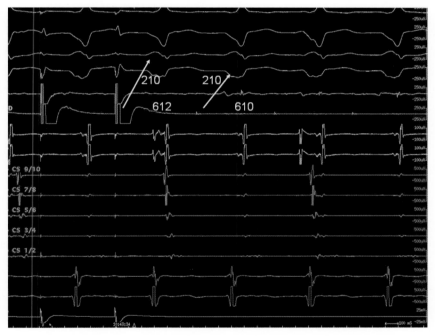

Figure 65.4 Transient entrainment from the distal electrode pair of the ablation catheter on the epicardial surface. Note that the post-pacing interval (612 ms) is similar to the VT cycle length (610 ms) with no change in the surface QRS morphology. The stimulus-to-QRS interval of 210 ms (arrow) during rapid pacing is identical to the local electrogram-to-QRS interval at the pacing site (arrow) indicating that the pacing site was located within the slowly conducting zone of the reentrant circuit.

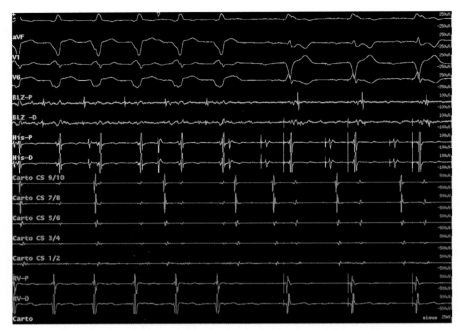

Figure 65.5   Termination of VT by the application of irrigated RF current (40 W) at the site of entrainment noted in Figures 65.3 and 65.4. Note that the VT slows before termination.

CHAPTER 66

Substrate modification in hemodynamically unstable infarct-related ventricular tachycardia

Kevin J. Makati, MD *& N. A. Mark Estes III,* MD

Clinical vignette

A 49-year-old male who had large anteroseptal ST elevation myocardial infarction (MI) and ventricular fibrillation arrest several months ago. A catheterization at that time showed a complete occlusion of the left anterior descending artery and the right coronary artery requiring emergent coronary artery bypass grafting. Because of his large infarction and poor results of bypass surgery, he was referred for consideration of heart transplantation. An implantable cardioverter defibrillator (ICD) was implanted during the interim period and he experienced multiple runs of poorly tolerated sustained ventricular tachycardia (VT) with several different morphologies despite multiple antiarrhythmic agents. He has had multiple ICD discharges due to sustained monomorphic VT. He was referred for catheter ablation of his VT.

Electrophysiology study and ablation

The patient was brought to the electrophysiology lab for substrate modification of the left ventricle. A voltage map of the left ventricle was constructed

Electroanatomical Mapping, 1st edition. Edited by A. Al-Ahmad, D. Callans, H. Hsia and A. Natale. © 2008 Blackwell Publishing, ISBN: 9781405157025.

revealing areas of dense scar along the anteroseptum surrounded by myocardium of variable electrical function (Figure 66.1). The maximum and minimum voltages were adjusted to maximally detect true scar from partially conducting areas of

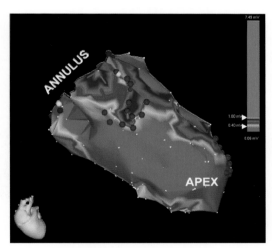

Figure 66.1 Electroanatomic map of left ventricle in right anterior oblique (RAO) projection. The red areas represent dense scar, defined as R-wave amplitudes less than 0.4 mV. Normal myocardium is represented by the color purple, defined as R-wave amplitudes greater than 1.0 mV. Myocardium with mixed functionality is represented as the color spectrum in between red and purple. Dense scar is noted over the anteroseptum. A site showing isolated diastolic potential (IDP) is labeled with a pink tag. Ablation lesions were placed connecting dense scar with the mitral annulus.

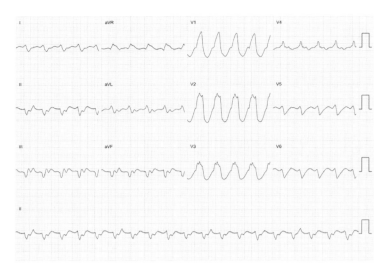

Figure 66.2 A 12-lead electro-cardiogram showing one of several clinical relevant unstable VTs with a right bundle branch block morphology and northwest axis in the frontal plane.

tissue. Mapping along an isthmus separating the infarct zone incited a VT closely resembling one of the clinically relevant tachycardias labeled with a pink tag in Figure 66.1. Pace-mapping over the inferior aspect of the left ventricle showed a very good morphologic match of the clinical tachycardia (Figure 66.2) and labeled with pink tags (Figures 66.3 and 66.4). Mapping along the infarct shows more fractionated electrograms with prolonged stimulus-to-QRS intervals that were targeted for ablation (Figure 66.5). Isolated diastolic potentials (IDPs) are noted during VT suggesting participation of the local myocardium in the VT circuit (Figure 66.6). Ablation targeting IDPs successfully terminated one of the clinical tachycardias. Lesions were then placed connecting areas of dense scar to the mitral annulus as well as in areas of complex fractionated electrograms. No further VT could be induced using standard programmed electrical stimulation protocols. The patient was discharged off antiarrhythmic medications without further ventricular arrhythmias. Electroanatomic mapping of unstable VT offers an alternative to classical entrainment mapping of VT, which requires induction and maintenance of the arrhythmia long enough to perform diagnostic maneuvers confirming the identity of participating circuits. Several approaches have been demonstrated including pace-mapping, identification of gross anatomic isthmuses with bipolar voltage mapping, and elimination of fractionated potentials that may

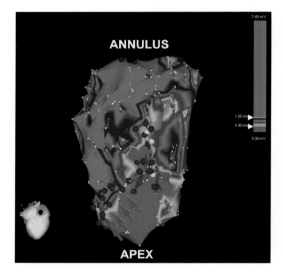

Figure 66.3 Electroanatomic map of left ventricle in inferior projection. The map definition is as described in Figure 66.1. Green arrows indicate areas of complex fractionated electrograms with prolonged stimulus to electrogram intervals. Pink tags indicate areas of IDPs.

be critical to tachycardia maintenance. Prolonged, paced stimulus-to-QRS at complex fractionated electrograms sites has been suggested to represent myocardium participating in reentrant circuits and, therefore successful ablation sites. The location an IDP is observed suggests that the underlying myocardium is within a reentrant circuit and marks a potentially successful ablation site.

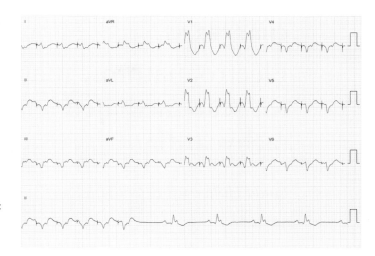

Figure 66.4 Pace-mapping in the left ventricle showing a match with the clinical tachycardia. Note the prolonged stimulus-to-QRS interval.

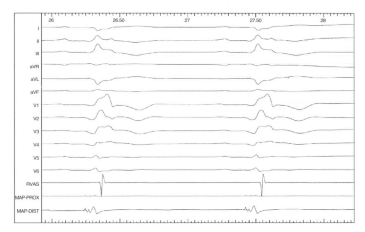

Figure 66.5 Complex fractionated potentials. Electrograms from the mapping catheter (MAP-DIST) around infarct border zones were complex, fractionated, and prolonged. Lesions were placed in these areas.

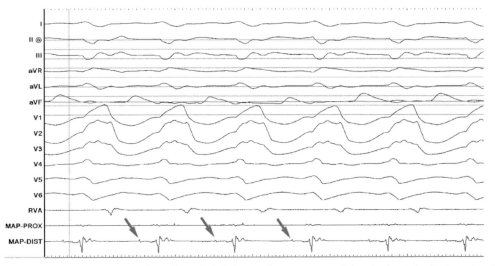

Figure 66.6 IDPs were noted during the tachycardia in isthmuses between scar and the mitral annulus. Lesions placed during the tachycardia resulted in termination.

CHAPTER 67

Electroanatomic mapping for scar-mediated left ventricular tachycardia

Linda Huffer, MD *& William Stevenson,* MD

Clinical vignette

The patient is an octogenarian with a history of three-vessel coronary artery disease, old anterior myocardial infarction, heart failure, and recent upgrade of a dual-chamber implantable cardioverter defibrillator (ICD) to a biventricular device. He presented with ventricular tachycardia (VT) storm despite antiarrhythmic therapy including amiodarone, mexilitine, and sotalol.

Device interrogation revealed approximately 60 episodes of pace-terminable monomorphic VT, cycle length (CL) 510 ms, which occurred in the eight days prior to admission. Left ventricular pacing was turned off to eliminate any possible proarrhythmic effect. Sustained monomorphic VT recurred during hospitalization consistent with his clinical tachycardia (Figure 67.1).

A cardiac catheterization demonstrated a 90% mid-left anterior descending artery stenosis,

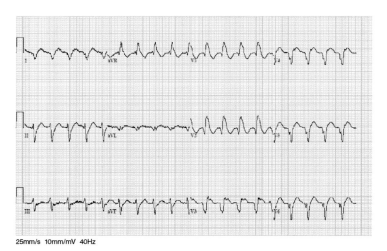

25mm/s 10mm/mV 40Hz

Figure 67.1 Clinical VT, 12-lead electrogram (EGM). VT QRS complexes demonstrate a right bundle branch block configuration, superiorly directed extreme right frontal plane axis, and precordial transition at V3, rate 116 bpm (CL 517 ms). This morphology suggests a left ventricular origin with a possible inferior and apical exit.

Electroanatomical Mapping, 1st edition. Edited by
A. Al-Ahmad, D. Callans, H. Hsia and A. Natale.
© 2008 Blackwell Publishing, ISBN: 9781405157025.

proximal occlusion of the left circumflex artery, and nonobstructive disease of the mid right coronary artery. A PET-CT (Dipyridamole-stress Rubidium-82) demonstrated a large, fixed anterior defect consistent with trans-mural scar in the mid left anterior descending artery distribution. Echocardiography revealed a left ventricular ejection fraction of 30–35% with mid-to-distal anteroseptal, apical, and posterior akinesis with anterior and anterolateral hypokinesis and no left ventricular thrombus.

Electrophysiology study and ablation

Baseline tracings showed sinus rhythm with first degree AV block, left bundle branch block, prolonged AH interval (150 ms), and a normal HV interval (54 ms). Programmed ventricular stimulation from the right ventricular apex induced two different monomorphic VTs. The first VT, which terminated spontaneously, had a CL of 360 ms, a right bundle branch block configuration, superiorly directed frontal plane axis, and a precordial transition at V4 substantially different from the patient's spontaneous tachycardia. The second induced sustained monomorphic VT (Figure 67.2)

had a CL and morphology consistent with his spontaneous, clinical tachycardia and was easily terminated with burst pacing delivered from the right ventricular apex.

A left ventricular electroanatomic map was then obtained in sinus rhythm using the CARTO™ system and a saline irrigated mapping and ablation catheter (Thermocool; Biosense Webster, Inc.). VT substrate was delineated by pace-mapping and annotating sites of fractionation, late systolic potentials, and low-voltage (<1.5 mV) scar. Unipolar pacing at 10 mA/2 ms was utilized for pace-mapping and determination of electrically unexcitable scar (EUS) that were marked as scar (gray regions). The clinical VT was re-induced during catheter manipulation in the left ventricle. The tachycardia was stable and regular allowing entrainment to be assessed from selected sites as the electroanatomic map was created. Outer loop (Figure 67.3a and b), remote bystander (Figure 67.4), and exit (Figure 67.5a and b) sites were identified. RF ablation was applied at a site with a low-voltage isolated diastolic potential (Figure 67.6) consistent with an exit by entrainment mapping. Tachycardia terminated during ablation (Figure 67.7). Additional ablation was then applied in sinus rhythm at sites of isolated late

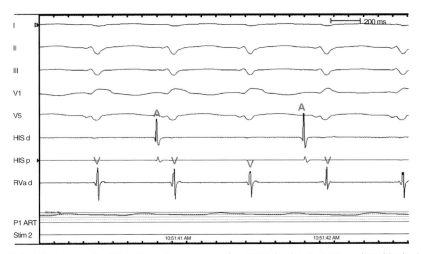

Figure 67.2 Clinical VT, intracardiac EGMs. From the top are surface EGMs leads I, II, III, V1, and V5, bipolar intracardiac EGMs recorded from the His catheter (proximal, distal), and RV apex (distal), and the femoral arterial pressure waveform. This tachycardia, with a CL approximately from 500 ms to 520 ms, was easily induced with ventricular programmed stimulation and catheter manipulation in the left ventricle. Intracardiac EGMs demonstrate AV dissociation consistent with a diagnosis of VT. The surface EGM morphology was consistent with the patient's clinical tachycardia (see Figure 67.1). Note the stable femoral arterial pressure of 90–100/40–50 mmHg that allowed for entrainment and activation mapping.

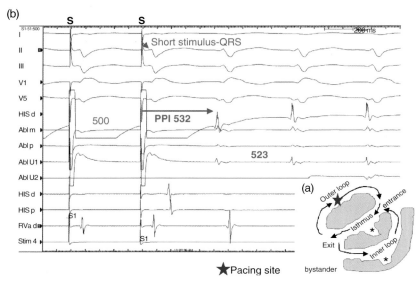

Figure 67.3 Entrainment from an outer loop site. From the top are surface EGMs leads I, II, III, V1, and V5, bipolar intracardiac EGMs recorded from the ablation catheter (distal, mid, and proximal) unipolar EGMs recorded from the ablation catheter (U1, U2), and bipolar EGMs recorded from the His catheter (proximal, distal), and RV apex (distal). The last two stimuli (S) of a train at a CL of 500 ms are shown followed by continuation of the VT at 523 ms. The stimuli entrain VT but change the QRS morphology consistent with entrainment with manifest fusion. The postpacing interval (PPI), measured from the last pacing stimulus to diastolic electrical activity is approximately the tachycardia CL (PPI-VTCL <30 ms), consistent with a reentry circuit site. During entrainment, the interval from the stimulus–QRS onset is short (20 ms). These findings are consistent with entrainment from an outer loop site (a). The schematic representation shows a theoretical VT circuit within inexcitable infarct scar. (b) This figure shows the 12-lead ECG during entrainment. Manifest fusion is most evident in surface leads V3 and V4 (blue arrows) where differences in the QRS complex notches are seen (arrows).

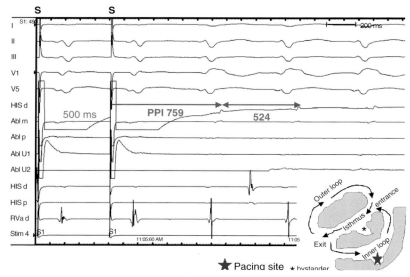

Figure 67.4 Entrainment from remote bystander site. Tracings are as in the figure. The last two stimuli (S) of a train at a CL of 500 ms are shown followed by continuation of the VT at 524 ms. During tachycardia, pacing accelerates the QRS complexes to the pacing CL with a markedly different morphology compared to the clinical tachycardia, consistent with fusion. The PPI is 759 ms, which is substantially longer than the tachycardia CL. These findings are consistent with entrainment from a remote bystander site.

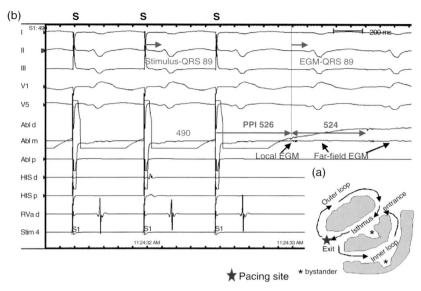

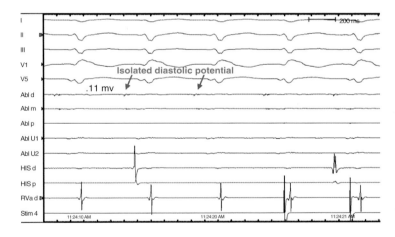

Figure 67.5 Entrainment from the VT exit. Tracings are as in Figure 67.4. The last three stimuli (S) of a train at a CL of 490 ms are shown followed by continuation of the VT at 525 ms. The stimuli entrain VT without altering the QRS complex, consistent with entrainment with concealed fusion (ECF). The PPI is approximately equal to the VT CL, consistent with a reentry circuit site. During entrainment, the interval from the stimulus–QRS onset is 89 ms. This interval is equal to the EGM–QRS interval and is 17% of the VT TCL (<30% of VT CL). These findings are consistent with entrainment from an exit site (a). The 12-lead surface EKG demonstrating ECF is shown in (b). The local and far-field EGMs are labeled. The pacing stimuli capture the local EGM. Therefore, it is not visible during the drive train while the far-field EGMs are visible both during entrainment and upon termination of pacing.

Figure 67.6 Isolated diastolic potential at successful ablation site. Tracings are as in Figure 67.4. A low-voltage (0.11 mV) isolated diastolic potential was present at the exit site (Figure 67.5a) during tachycardia. These potentials are generated by depolarization through isolated muscle fibers in scar. They are often present in a narrow isthmus in the reentry circuit at sites associated with successful ablation.

potentials in a channel between regions of EUS (Figure 67.8). Electroanatomical substrate and activation maps are shown in Figures 67.9 and 67.10. Ablation was continued until this region was rendered electrically unexcitable. Ventricular burst pacing and programmed extrastimula-tion was then repeated with up to double extrastimuli at two CLs inducing brief (4.8 s) runs of polymorphic VT.

The patient remained arrhythmia free throughout the remainder of his hospital stay and was discharged on amiodarone 200 mg once a day and Toprol XL 100 mg once a day. He remained free of arrhythmias as of his last evaluation 6 weeks after ablation.

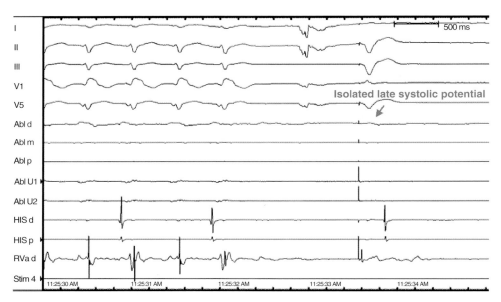

Figure 67.7 VT termination during ablation. Tracings are as in Figure 67.4. VT terminated without a premature ventricular contraction approximately 38 s after the onset of the first ablation lesion at the exit. The last beat in the tracing is a ventricular paced complex that demonstrates an isolated late systolic potential consistent with slowed conduction.

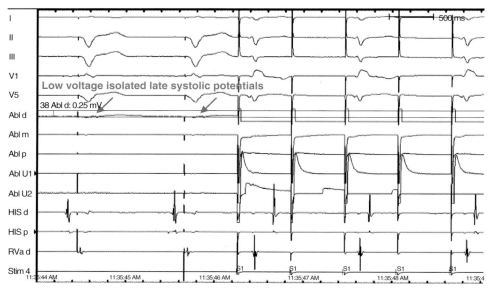

Figure 67.8 Isolated late systolic potentials. Tracings are as in Figure 67.4. Pacing from the distal ablation catheter with 2:1 capture is shown in a region with slowed conduction manifest by very low-voltage isolated late systolic potentials. This site was adjacent to the initial ablation lesion. Ablation was applied at this site and through a channel between regions of EUS until the area was rendered electrically unexcitable with unipolar pacing at 10 mA/2 ms pulse width.

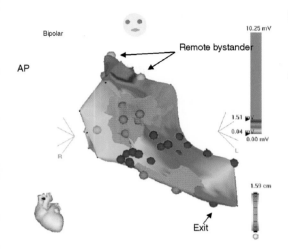

Remote bystander: yellow; ablation lesions: red;
EUS: gray; outer loop: blue

Figure 67.9 Electroanatomic substrate map: AP view. The voltage map was constructed during sinus rhythm. Areas with EGM voltage <0.04 mV are in red. Areas with normal EGM voltage of >1.5 mV are in purple. A large region of low voltage is evident in the anterior, septal, and apical left ventricle consistent with prior myocardial infarction. EUS is shown in gray. Exit, outer loop, and bystander sites identified during entrainment mapping are annotated. Ablation sites are marked with dark red circles.

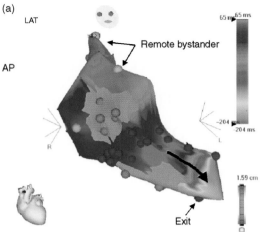

Remote bystander: yellow; ablation lesions: red; EUS;
gray; outer loop: blue

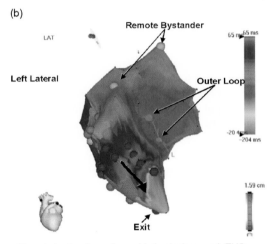

Remote bystander: yellow; ablation lesions: red; EUS;
gray; outer loop: blue

Figure 67.10 VT activation map: AP view (a) and left lateral view (b). Activation proceeds from red, to yellow, to green, to blue, to purple as the wave front proceeds to the exit region, then superiorly and inferiorly along the infarct margin. Just proximal to the exit, earliest activation meets latest activation, characteristic of a reentry circuit. The complete circuit was not defined. Note the activation time color coded from −204 ms to + 65 ms sum to 269 ms, approximately 52% of the VT CL. Tachycardia termination, however, was achieved with ablation at the exit. The entire reentry circuit does not, therefore, need to be delineated with this approach when a desirable target site is identified. Exit, outer loop, and bystander sites identified during entrainment mapping are annotated. Ablation sites are marked with dark red circles.

CHAPTER 68

Ventricular tachycardia, endocardial, and epicardial mapping

Jonathan Sussman, MD

Clinical vignette

A 32-year-old female without prior cardiac or medical history developed palpitations. Holter monitoring revealed self-terminating episodes of sustained ventricular tachycardia (VT). Subsequent testing included: an echocardiogram with infero-lateral hypokineses and overall left ventricular ejection fraction of 40–45%; nuclear stress test that showed an inferolateral scar; and cardiac catheterization that revealed an anomalous small left circumflex arising from the right aortic cusp, but no other significant coronary disease.

During her hospital stay, she had frequent, self-limited episodes of VT with two different morphologies. A cardiac MRI revealed areas of wall thinning in the inferior and anterolateral walls. Areas of epicardial and mid-myocardial delayed enhancement were observed within the anterior interventricular septum, as well as basal, mid, and apical septum. Large confluent area epicardial and mid-myocardial delayed enhancement in inferior septum extending to inferior and inferolateral walls from mid-cavity to apex was also noted. MRI findings were felt not to reflect any vascular distribution and to represent a nonischemic cardiomyopathy or myocarditis.

Electrophysiology study and ablation

Two morphologies of VT were seen, matching her clinical arrhythmias (Figures 68.1 and 68.2). The first occurred spontaneously; the second had a stuttering onset after programmed stimulation. Endocardial mapping revealed no areas of fractionated electrograms, diastolic activity during VT, or late potentials during sinus rhythm. In addition, only a very small area of low-amplitude electrograms was seen at the basal anteroseptum (Figure 68.3). Endocardial pace-mapping from the infero-lateral wall resulted in a marginal QRS match. Epicardial mapping revealed more extensive areas of low voltage overlying the right ventricle, inter-ventricular septum, and inferolateral left ventricle (Figure 68.4). Late potentials at the inferolateral wall further suggested the presence of scar, rather than overlying epicardial fat. Pace-maps closely matching both clinical VTs were seen in the area of scar, suggesting an epicardial site of origin (Figure 68.5). However, diaphragmatic stimulation was seen during pacing throughout this area, and ablation was therefore deferred to avoid risking phrenic nerve injury.

Electroanatomical Mapping, 1st edition. Edited by
A. Al-Ahmad, D. Callans, H. Hsia and A. Natale.
© 2008 Blackwell Publishing, ISBN: 9781405157025.

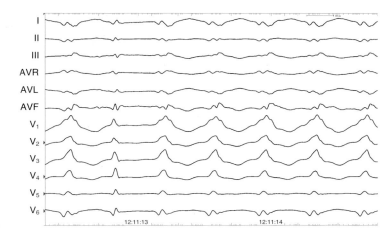

Figure 68.1   VT 1 with a right bundle, right superior axis (RBRS) QRS morphology occurring spontaneously during mapping.

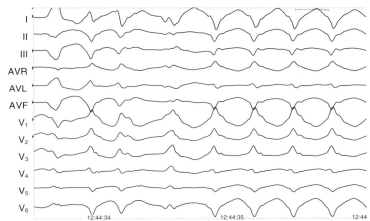

Figure 68.2   VT 2 with a similar RBRS QRS morphology as VT 1, induced with programmed stimulation.

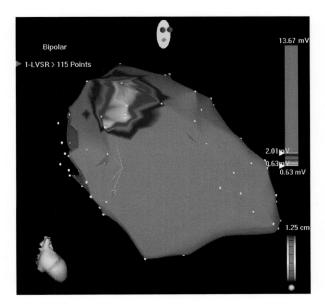

Figure 68.3   Left ventricular endocardial voltage map, right anterior oblique (RAO) projection. Purple colored areas represent normal endocardium (amplitude ≥2.0 mV) with scarred area depicted as red-yellow color (amplitude < 2.0 mV). Only a very small area of low-amplitude electrograms was seen at the basal septum.

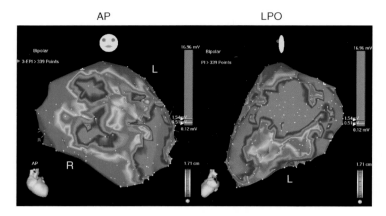

Figure 68.4　Epicardial voltage maps in AP and left posterior oblique (LPO) projections. The voltage criteria were similar to Figure 68.3 with purple color represent normal endocardium (amplitude ≥1.5 mV) and dense scar depicted as red (amplitude <0.5 mV). The border zone (amplitude 0.5–1.5 mV) is defined as areas with the intermediate color gradient.

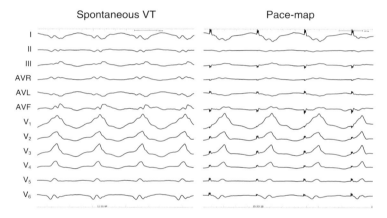

Figure 68.5　Best pace-map for VT 1 from epicardium.

CHAPTER 69

Endocardial and epicardial mapping for ventricular tachycardia in the setting of myocarditis

David Callans, MD, FACC, FHRS

Clinical vignette

A 50-year-old man had a course of viral myocarditis, resulting in severe left ventricular dysfunction (ejection fraction between 10% and 15%). He underwent implantable cardioverter defibrillator (ICD) placement for primary prevention. Several years later, he developed uniform sustained right bundle, right inferior (RBRI) axis ventricular tachycardia (VT) (cycle length 440 ms) that was refractory to antiarrhythmic drugs and resulted in recurrent ICD shocks. He was referred for catheter ablation.

Electrophysiology study and ablation

The clinical VT was easily induced and EnSite Array mapping of the LV was performed (Figure 69.1). On close examination, this map demonstrates a very wide, diffuse area of earliest endocardial activation. The point of activation of the unipolar recordings begins after the onset of the surface QRS. Finally, pace-mapping from the site of earliest endocardial activation did not match the QRS morphology of the VT. All of these facts support the diagnosis of an epicardial site of VT origin. He returned on another day for endocardial and epicardial contact mapping. Endocardial voltage mapping demonstrated an area of scar in the area of earliest endocardial activation, and several RF lesions were delivered to the edge of the scar without effect (Figure 69.2). Epicardial activation mapping demonstrated much earlier sites and entrainment mapping proved participation in the VT circuit. Epicardial ablation resulted in the prompt termination of the tachycardia. Note that the epicardial location of the VT circuit is not directly opposite the site of earliest activation on the endocardium (Figure 69.3).

Electroanatomical Mapping, 1st edition. Edited by
A. Al-Ahmad, D. Callans, H. Hsia and A. Natale.

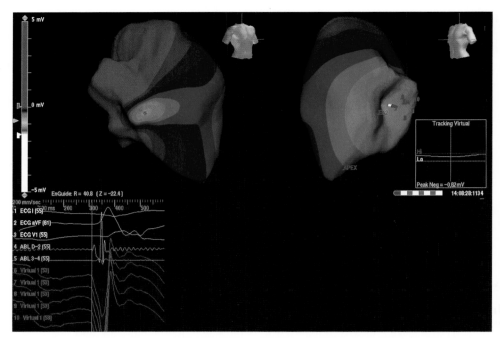

Figure 69.1   ESI mapping of the LV during VT using the noncontact array demonstrated an elatively diffuse area of earliest endocardial activation.

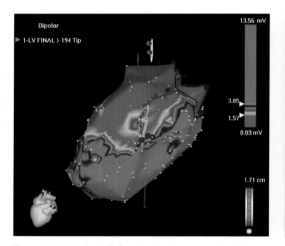

Figure 69.2   Endocardial contact voltage map showing an area of scar near the area of earliest activation. Scar was defined as areas with abnormal local bipolar electrogram voltage of less than 1.57 mV.

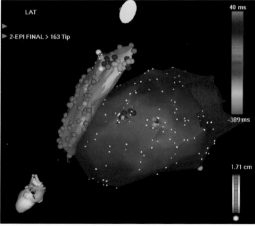

Figure 69.3   Epicardial activation map showing the areas early activation.

CHAPTER 70

Multiple left ventricular basal ventricular tachycardias in a patient with dilated cardiomyopathy

Jason Jacobsen, MD

Clinical vignette

A 69-year-old man with a history of nonischemic dilated cardiomyopathy and implantable cardioverter defibrillator (ICD) implantation presented with multiple ICD shocks for ventricular tachycardia (VT). He had been on multiple antiarrhythmic drugs in the past without effect. He underwent electrophysiologic study (EPS) at another institution prior to transfer for ablative therapy. Multiple VT morphologies were induced with programmed stimulation.

Electrophysiology study and ablation

The patient was transferred and underwent an EPS. Six VT (Figure 70.1) morphologies were induced, but the procedure was aborted due to pericardial tamponade. Limited activation and pace-mapping localized all VTs to the basal LV either adjacent to the aortic valve or the anterior mitral annulus.

One week later, a second ablation session was undertaken. Owing to the morphologic characteristics (time to peak of R wave >55% of the QRS duration in the precordial leads; QS in lead I) of some of the VTs induced at the first session,

Electroanatomical Mapping, 1st edition. Edited by A. Al-Ahmad, D. Callans, H. Hsia and A. Natale. © 2008 Blackwell Publishing, ISBN: 9781405157025.

epicardial (in addition to endocardial) access was obtained. Voltage mapping with CARTO™ revealed a small basal anteroseptal endocardial scar and a large peri-annular epicardial low-voltage area (Figure 70.2). Another six VT morphologies were induced (Figure 70.3). These were similar to the VTs induced at the first session but morphologically distinct. One of these VTs was mapped to the endocardial scar and ablated there (Figure 70.4a). The rest were mapped to the epicardial scar between the anteroseptal and lateral borders (Figure 70.4b). A linear set of RF lesions was applied to the epicardial scar connecting these areas (Figure 70.5). Coronary angiography was performed to assure adequate distances from the major epicardial coronary arteries (>10 mm). Over the next few days, the patient developed recurrent ICD shocks for a new, but morphologically similar VTs.

The patient underwent repeat EPS approximately one week later for endocardial mapping and ablation. Endocardial voltage mapping again revealed a small anteroseptal scar. Five new, but similar, VT morphologies were induced (Figure 70.6). The exit site for one dominant VT was located in the endocardial scar by entrainment mapping. Pace-mapping within the scar also resulted in good QRS match for two other VTs at the anterior annular region in scar border zone (Figure 70.7). A linear set of RF lesions was applied across the basal LV from just lateral to the His to the anterolateral annulus, matching the epicardial lesion set from the previous ablation session (Figure 70.7).

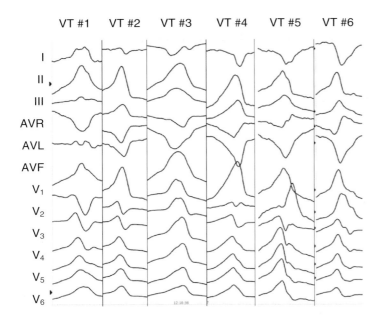

VT #1   VT #2   VT #3   VT #4   VT #5   VT #6

I
II
III
AVR
AVL
AVF
V₁
V₂
V₃
V₄
V₅
V₆

Figure 70.1   The six VT morphologies induced at the first ablation session. Notice the progression from left bundle branch block (LBBB) to right bundle branch block (RBBB) morphology with an inferior axis in all. The early transition in the precordial leads suggests a basal origin for each VT.

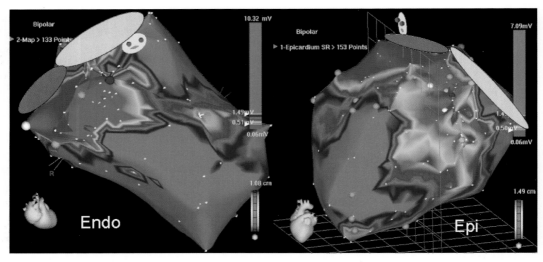

Figure 70.2   Endocardial (Endo) and epicardial (Epi) LV voltage maps obtained during the second ablation session. Note the basal, peri-annular location of the low-voltage areas. Normal voltage (1.5 mV) is indicated as purple, scar (<0.5 mV) as red, and border zone (0.5–1.49 mV) as yellow to blue. Gray ovals indicate the mitral valve, and blue ovals indicate the aortic valve.

Programmed stimulation failed to induce any clinical basal LV VT. The patient had no further VT episodes for the remainder of his hospitalization and noninvasive programmed stimulation via his defibrillator prior to discharge did not induce any VT with a morphology consistent with a basal LV origin.

This case illustrates the peri-annular location of scar and VT site of origin in patients with dilated cardiomyopathy, often with a preponderance of scar in the epicardium. Although 17 different VT morphologies were induced, they all were quite similar and originated near the annular LV from low-voltage areas. Attempts at entrainment

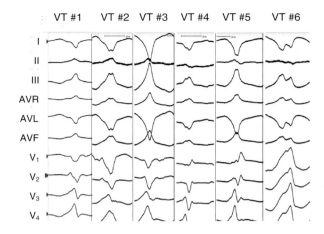

Figure 70.3 The six VT morphologies induced at the second ablation session. The morphologies were similar but distinct from the first set of induced VTs (Figure 70.1).

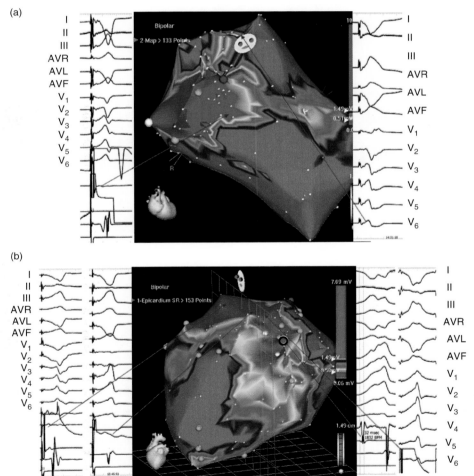

Figure 70.4 (a) Two endocardial pace-map sites. The pace-map on the left (Left bundle, left inferior axis (LBRI) QRS morphology) is a perfect match for one of the VTs (VT #2) and ablation was performed. The pace-map on the right resembles another of the VTs, but is not perfect. (b) Three epicardial pace-map sites and the local electrogram (EGM) during the predominant VT (VT #6) (green dot). The EGM–QRS interval at the green dot is consistent with an exit site of this VT. All three VTs were mapped to the epicardial scar between the anteroseptal and lateral borders.

were often thwarted by termination or changing of morphologies. "Segmental isolation" of the annular region from septum to lateral wall, both from the endo- and epicardium was required to render this patient noninducible. Although it was not possible to map all VTs during tachycardia (or verify their mechanisms), the abnormal myocardium at the LV base appears to be the underlying substrate for scar-based reentry VTs in this patient.

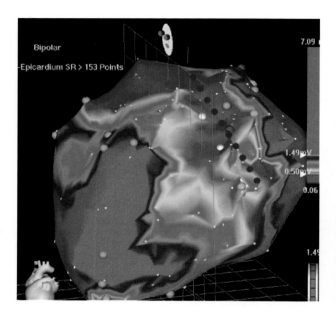

Figure 70.5 Linear ablation superimposed on an epicardial voltage map. The epicardial ablation lesion set (red dots) was designed to run parallel to the annular region within the scar to transect good pace-map and activation sites while staying 10 mm from the coronaries arteries.

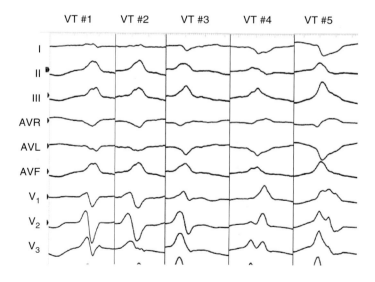

Figure 70.6 The five VT morphologies induced at the third ablation session. Note the similarities to the first and second set of VTs.

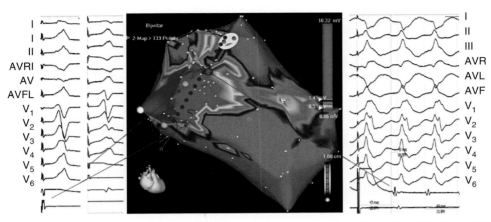

Figure 70.7 Linear ablation superimposed on an endocardial voltage map. Entrainment mapping of the dominant VT showed concealed fusion and an EGM–QRS interval consistent with an exit site (green dot). Pace-mapping within the scar also resulted in good QRS match for two other VTs to the anterior annular region in scar border zone. The line of red dots indicates the ablation lesion set starting from just above the His (yellow dot in the blue circle) to the anterolateral mitral annulus, matching the epicardial lesion set from the previous ablation session.

CHAPTER 71

Epicardial ventricular tachycardia in a patient with nonischemic cardiomyopathy

Rupa Bala, MD

Clinical vignette

The patient is a 78-year-old male with a history of nonischemic cardiomyopathy, low ejection fraction of 30%, and biventricular implantable cardioverter defibrillator (ICD). He presented with palpitations, presyncope, and recurrent ventricular tachycardia (VT) with multiple shocks for electrophysiology study and ablation.

Electrophysiology study and ablation

Electrophysiology study induced multiple VTs. Extensive endocardial and epicardial mapping were performed using the three-dimensional CARTO™ system. Figure 71.1 is an example of a right bundle, right inferior (RBRI) axis VT. Mid-diastolic potentials were present and entrainment mapping identified isthmus and exit sites (Figure 71.2). Coronary angiogram was performed to ascertain the locations of the coronary arteries (Figure 71.3) and the VT was terminated in the epicardium with a single RF lesion (Figure 71.4). There was a perfect pace-map at the epicardial site of termination (Figure 71.5).

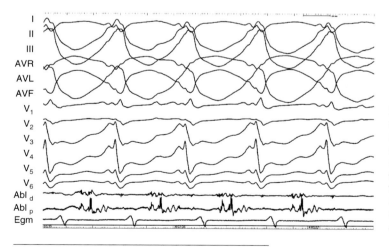

Figure 71.1 RBRI VT. Mid-diastolic potentials (arrows) were noted in the basal, anterolateral epicardium during epicardial mapping of this VT. Note the ECG features suggestive of epicardial VT: QS pattern in lead I, slurred upstroke, and pattern break in V1–V3 with a R–S complex <1 in V2.

Electroanatomical Mapping, 1st edition. Edited by
A. Al-Ahmad, D. Callans, H. Hsia and A. Natale.
© 2008 Blackwell Publishing, ISBN: 9781405157025.

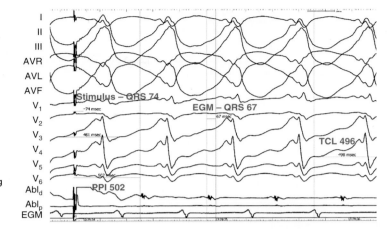

Figure 71.2 Entrainment mapping is used to identify an exit site for the RBRI VT on the basal, anterolateral epicardium.

Left coronary artery angiogram

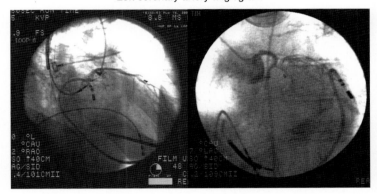

Figure 71.3 Prior to radiofrequency ablation, an angiogram is performed. The ablation catheter is positioned in the epicardium at the isthmus exit site with mid-diastolic potentials.

VT Termination with epicardial

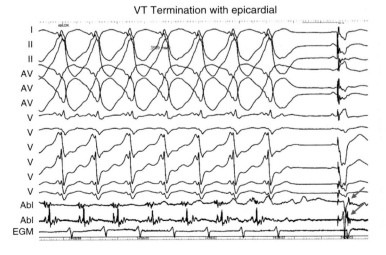

Figure 71.4 The VT terminates in less than 4 s in the epicardium at this site. Note the late potentials on the ablation catheter (arrows) on the paced beat after tachycardia termination.

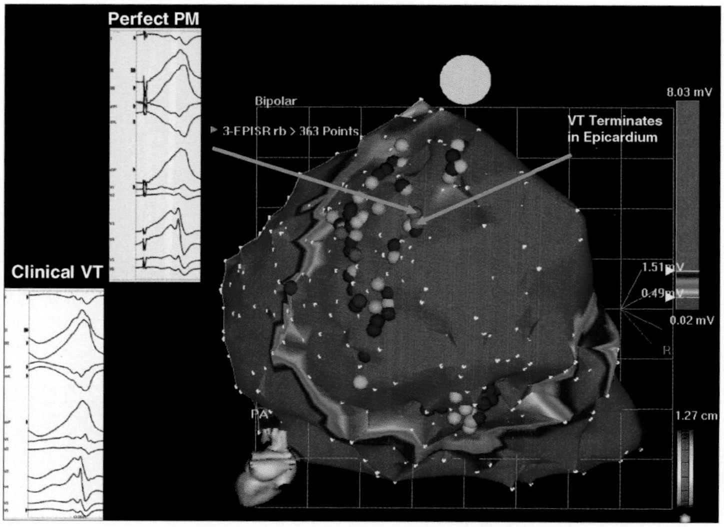

Figure 71.5   Electroanatomical voltage map of basal, anterolateral epicardium is shown with the site of VT termination and perfect pace-map.

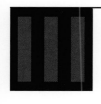

PART III
Tips and tricks

CHAPTER 72

Three-dimensional mapping and navigation with the EnSite Array and NavX system

Craig A. Swygman, & Blair D. Halperin, MD

Introduction

Mapping of cardiac arrhythmias has evolved from maneuvering nondeflectable quadripolar catheters under fluoroscopic guidance to the use of computerized three-dimensional mapping and navigation systems with minimal fluoroscopy. Techniques initially utilized sequential point-by-point mapping, whereas current mapping systems allow simultaneous assessment of electrogram information from multiple electrodes and catheters. Conventional mapping typically required sustained tachycardia or frequent ectopy; newer mapping systems allow single-beat mapping for infrequent ectopy and identification of arrhythmogenic substrates without inducing tachycardia.

The EnSite System (St. Jude Medical, St. Paul, MN) was introduced in the United States in the late 1990s [1]. The system has two technologies that can facilitate electrophysiologic mapping and ablation procedures. The EnSite Array catheter and computer-based system allows for noncontact mapping of conduction through a cardiac chamber in a single cycle of the tachycardia. The EnSite NavX system allows for three-dimensional graphic representation of any cardiac chamber and catheter navigation using a combination of cutaneous patches and intracardiac catheters. The NavX system can perform isochronal activation mapping and display electrogram voltage for the identification of

arrhythmogenic substrates, such as scar in patients with prior myocardial infarction.

Both the Array and NavX systems can assist in mapping of complex tachyarrhythmias and allow for catheter navigation with limited fluoroscopic exposure for patient or physician.

EnSite Array catheter and system

Conventional catheter-based mapping is limited by the number of sites that the operator sequentially positions the mapping catheter. This limitation is especially problematic in patients with nonsustained tachycardia, hemodynamically unstable tachycardias, or rhythms that are difficult to induce. The EnSite Array mapping system is a computerized system that creates three-dimensional electroanatomical maps without the need for point-by-point contact electrograms. A noncontact balloon catheter creates virtual unipolar electrograms using a mathematical inverse solution to estimate the electrical potentials.

The EnSite System consists of a 9-Fr multielectrode-array catheter mounted on a 7.5-mL balloon, amplifiers, and a computer work station. There are 64 insulated 0.003-in. diameter wires around the circumference of the balloon. Each wire has a 0.025-in. break in the insulation that serves as the unipolar electrode. The array size, when inflated, is 1.8×4.6 cm. The array catheter is positioned in the cardiac chamber over a 0.035-in. guide wire placed in the lumen of the balloon catheter. The balloon is expanded and deployed by injection of a 50% mixture of contrast media and saline.

Electroanatomical Mapping, 1st edition. Edited by
A. Al-Ahmad, D. Callans, H. Hsia and A. Natale.
© 2008 Blackwell Publishing, ISBN: 9781405157025.

The system has the capability of localizing any conventional electrode catheter by emitting a low-current locator signal at 5.68 kHz from the catheter tip electrode and "sensed" by two ring electrodes located on the array. The locator signal is processed to create a three-dimensional model of the cardiac chamber while a "roving" catheter is "swept" throughout the chamber. With the multielectrode array in position in the chamber, far-field potentials are recorded, amplified, digitized, sampled at 1.2 kHz, and filtered at 0.1–300 Hz. The resulting signals are used to create 3360 virtual unipolar electrograms. The computed isopotential or voltage data from the virtual electrograms are displayed on a three-dimensional endocardial map. Isopotential or isochronal activation maps can be reconstructed from a single cycle of the tachycardia because of simultaneous signal acquisition.

Focal tachycardia

Mapping and ablation procedures for tachycardias that arise from a focal location, such as ectopic atrial tachycardia or right ventricular outflow tract ventricular tachycardia, usually have a high success rate. Ablation strategy involves targeting the site of earliest activation. Historically, conventional mapping consisted of one or two sequentially moving roving catheters throughout the area of interest until the site of earliest activation was found. Computer-based electroanatomical mapping and navigation systems have contributed significantly to the success of these procedures. Contact catheter mapping systems allow for cataloging of activation times at sequential anatomical locations. The EnSite Array system has several potential advantages over contact-based systems. Because of simultaneous acquisition of over 3000 electrograms, activation timing maps can be created from a single cycle of the tachycardia. This feature is especially advantageous for patients with nonsustained tachycardias, with infrequent atrial or ventricular ectopy, or whose rhythms are difficult to induce [2].

The technique for noncontact mapping involves the deployment of the multielectrode array in the cardiac chamber, creation of the anatomical geometry, and acquisition and processing of the virtual electrogram data. Global potential voltage maps are created from a single beat of the tachycardia. Activation can be tracked on the isopotential map

throughout the cycle to the onset of the tachycardia beat. Virtual electrodes are placed on the map to analyze the corresponding unipolar electrograms. The origin of the tachycardia is defined as the earliest site showing a QS pattern on the unipolar electrogram (Figure 72.1). The QS or negative potential represents activation away from the site of focal origin. Early sites with an rS pattern may represent foci that are epicardial in origin, or early activation sites in an adjacent structure (Figure 72.2). Isochronal maps can also be created, which represent the progression of activation throughout the chamber relative to a user-defined reference timing point. The EnSite System allows for a simplified display of an early activation site. This feature is called the "Find Early Activation" tool. The time cursor is placed at the onset of surface ECG activation, "Find Early Activation" is clicked with the mouse cursor, filtering is automatically adjusted, and the point of early activation is indicated on the map.

Several investigators have demonstrated and validated the EnSite Array system for mapping of atrial and ventricular tachycardias of focal origin. Higa *et al.* mapped and ablated 14 focal atrial tachycardias using the noncontact array catheter in 13 patients [3]. All tachycardia foci were located in the right atrium, with 57% along the crista terminalis. The EnSite System demonstrated the earliest site of activation, as well as the breakout sites and directions of preferential conduction, on the three-dimensional maps. Catheter ablation was successful both at the site of origin, as well as in the proximal portion of preferential conduction. Friedman *et al.* reported mapping of right ventricular outflow tract ventricular tachycardia using the EnSite noncontact system in 10 patients [4]. In 5 of 10 patients, only isolated ectopy or infrequent nonsustained tachycardia was present during the mapping procedure. Noncontact-guided ablation was acutely successful in 9 of 10 patients.

Reentrant tachycardia

The advent of three-dimensional systems has added greatly to the ability of electrophysiologists to successfully map and ablate complex reentrant tachycardias. Typical and atypical atrial flutter, as well as ventricular tachycardia in patients with a prior myocardial infarction, can be difficult reentrant arrhythmias to map using conventional

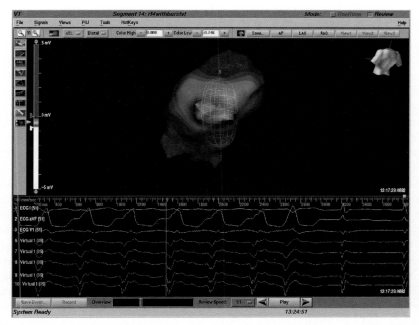

Figure 72.1 Noncontact isopotential map in patient with right ventricular outflow tract tachycardia. Caliper line on virtual electrograms is pre-QRS indicating early activation. Unipolar electrograms (6–10) show QS morphology, consistent with site of focal origin of the tachycardia.

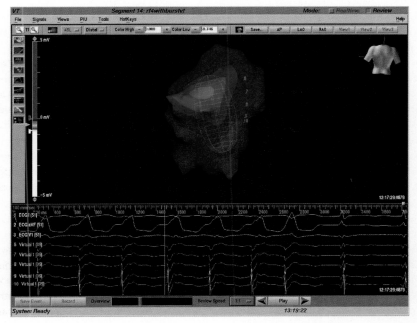

Figure 72.2 Noncontact isopotential map in the same patient as Figure 72.1. Note that the virtual electrograms (6–10) at a distance from the site of earliest activation show an rS electrogram morphology.

techniques. Entrainment techniques require a sustained arrhythmia, which can be difficult in the case of hemodynamically unstable ventricular tachycardia. Noncontact mapping allows for mapping of a single cycle of the tachycardia without the requirement of a sustained arrhythmia. Noncontact mapping has been used to confirm or demonstrate the anatomical location of a reentrant circuit. Because of global mapping capability, entire reentrant circuits can be demonstrated, including isthmus and exit locations. Klemm *et al.* compared noncontact identification of exit sites to contact maps of scar in 12 patients with ventricular tachycardia after myocardial infarction [5]. Exit sites identified by noncontact mapping were located within the border zone of the myocardial scar defined by scar voltage criteria. Owing to its ability to record from multiple sites simultaneously, noncontact mapping is able to identify gaps in previously placed linear lesion sets, such as in the cavotricuspid isthmus for typical atrial flutter. Schumacher *et al.* showed that noncontact maps could identify sites of conduction breaking through incomplete linear lesions [6].

The EnSite Array noncontact system allows for two ways of determining the location of the critical isthmus of slow conduction in reentrant arrhythmias, such as macroreentrant atrial flutter or ventricular tachycardia in patients with a prior myocardial infarction. The standard use of virtual electrogram data displayed on a three-dimensional map may be used for reentrant tachycardias, as previously described for focal tachycardias. The display can demonstrate the propagation of wave fronts, and locate areas with unipolar QS morphology. The unipolar QS electrogram that precedes the onset of the surface P wave or QRS for atrial or ventricular rhythms, respectively, is considered the source of activation from which the depolarizing wave front spreads to the rest of the chamber. This location is considered to be the exit site from the critical isthmus of slow conduction. Following the identification of the exit site, isthmus conduction can be traced back in time through the diastolic segment of the cardiac cycle. The earliest site of endocardial activation prior to the exit can be identified and marked on the anatomical geometry. Several investigators have published their experience using the EnSite Array for mapping and

ablation of reentrant tachycardias. Della Bella *et al.* reported their results in mapping of 21 hemodynamically unstable postinfarction ventricular tachycardias with the noncontact system [7]. The endocardial exit site was defined in 21/21 and the diastolic pathway was identified in 17/21 ventricular tachycardias.

The second component of the EnSite Array system, which that can be applied to the identification of critical substrates in reentrant tachycardias is an automated voltage program called "Dynamic Substrate Mapping" (DSM). The DSM software program is used in conjunction with the noncontact array and the unipolar virtual electrogram information. DSM is a fully automated program that can be used to characterize signals during electrical diastole. The program displays relative voltage information as a static color map, called a ratiometric map. Each color represents a ratio of the unipolar voltage at each point relative to the maximum negative unipolar voltage during a user-defined time range. The user places the DSM time calipers between two flutter waves for atrial rhythms and between two QRSs for ventricular tachycardia, that is, electrical diastole. The anatomical area with the greatest voltage during this interval should represent conduction through the critical isthmus or diastolic pathway. Investigators have demonstrated the utility of this tool for the mapping of substrate-mediated tachycardias [8].

The EnSite Array has several limitations in clinical practice. The balloon catheter can be difficult to deploy in some chambers, due to its size or elongated shape. In the right ventricular outflow tract, the balloon can be unstable and cause ventricular ectopy. This can make mapping of clinical ectopy challenging. The accuracy of the virtual electrogram information can be limited in large cardiac chambers. Investigators have validated the accuracy of noncontact mapping if the distance from the center of the balloon array is less than 4 cm [1,2]. At distances greater than 4 cm, low-amplitude signals may not be detected. Owing to the morphology of the balloon catheter, electrogram information from the polar ends of the array can be less reliable than data from the circumferential or transverse direction. A well-known limitation of unipolar mapping is the recording of far-field signals, which may make the identification of local activation difficult.

EnSite's capability to allow adjustment of the filtering of the signals can alleviate much of this problem.

EnSite NavX mapping and navigation

The NavX mapping and navigation system received Food and Drug Administration (FDA) approval in the United States in 2003. NavX uses conventional catheters and cutaneous patches to provide three-dimensional catheter tracking and mapping [9]. Three pairs of patches are placed along three orthogonal axes, comprising a three-dimensional coordinate system. A low-amplitude 5.7-kHz signal is emitted from the patches and received by catheters within the heart. Catheter location is determined by measuring the resulting electrical potential or field strength received by the catheters.

The system has several features that are useful in mapping and ablation procedures. The system has capabilities similar to conventional electrophysiology (EP) recording systems, including the display and recording of surface ECG and intracardiac electrograms. The system has the ability to display up to 12 catheters and a total of 64 electrodes on the three-dimensional map, thus allowing catheter navigation with reduced fluoroscopic imaging. The graphic display of multiple catheters can be especially useful in atrial fibrillation ablations, as catheters in the heart and esophagus can be visualized (Figure 72.3). The NavX system can track the location of conventional EP catheters as they are maneuvered within a cardiac chamber and a geometric model of the chamber can be created. Activation and voltage data can be acquired and displayed on the three-dimensional geometric model. Ablation lesions can be marked on the surface of the geometric model or as three-dimensional lesions if they are not adjacent to a created geometry. Three-dimensional CT or MRI images can be imported and displayed next to the created anatomical geometry, which can facilitate anatomically based ablation procedures. Several investigators have published their experience with NavX, showing a reduction in fluoroscopy times when compared with conventional mapping [10–14].

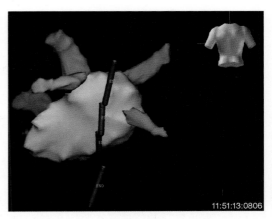

Figure 72.3   Posterior-anterior (PA) view of left atrial and pulmonary venous geometries created with NavX. Adjacent to the posterior wall of the left atrium are a series of "shadows" of a bipolar catheter placed in the esophagus

Geometry formation

The current approach for the mapping and ablation of some arrhythmias, such as atrial fibrillation and scar-mediated ventricular tachycardia, is anatomically based. The NavX system allows for the creation and display of multiple three-dimensional geometric representations of cardiac chambers. The creation of anatomical geometries is achieved by collecting three-dimensional locations as a catheter is maneuvered within a cardiac chamber. NavX geometries are created from a central point that is initially located at the tip electrode of the ablation catheter when geometry formation has begun. A volumetric "point-cloud" is collected out to the endocardial surface. Radiating spherically from the central point at 5° angles are three-dimensional, conical "bins." Each bin corresponds to a surface of the geometry, thus it has spherical coordinates. As points are collected, the bins are filled and updated. The displayed endocardial surface is determined by the points in each bin that are located at the farthest distance from the central point. The Geometry Detail feature allows the user to adjust the amount of interpolation between the point "bins." There is very little interpolation between bins with a "High" Geometry Detail setting; therefore, it is most useful with maps that have a high density of collected points. The "Advanced" setting allows for adjustment of the amount of interpolation and can be useful when relatively few points are collected. The user can assign specific points as endocardial surface points by using the "Locked Point" feature.

Prior to geometry creation, a positional reference must be determined. The displayed position of all catheters is relative to the location of the positional reference. The preferred positional reference is an intracardiac catheter that will remain in a stable location throughout the procedure. The coronary sinus catheter is often used because of its stability, especially when placed from the superior approach. Other catheter locations may also be used as the reference, such as right atrial appendage or a catheter in the esophagus for atrial fibrillation ablations. The original anatomic location of the reference catheter should be saved using the "Shadow" feature. The "Shadow" feature stores a static picture of the specific catheter position. During the procedure, the current reference catheter position can be compared to the saved "Shadow" position to assess for reference movement. The Enguide Responsiveness setting adjusts the visualized response speed between catheter motion and the navigation display. The Fast settings typically show all real-time catheter motion. The displayed catheter movement caused by respiratory and cardiac motion can be reduced by using the Moderate or Stable settings; however, there may be some delay in updating of the catheter displayed location. The effects of respiration on navigation can also be minimized by using the Respiration Compensation tool. Respiration Compensation collects a 12-s sample of measured impedance values from the skin patches. Respiration is identified by a gradual increase in the intrathoracic impedance. The system correlates the increase in impedance with a motion artifact on each displayed catheter. After Respiration Compensation has been completed, the system monitors the skin patches for the impedance pattern of respiration and gradually adjusts the displayed catheter positions to compensate in correlation with the degree of impedance change. Respiration Compensation may need to be re-collected during the procedure, for instance, after moving the catheter from one chamber to another, or when there is a significant change in breathing pattern.

An advantage of the NavX system is that any catheter can be utilized as the Active Enguide and used for creating geometry. Geometry formation

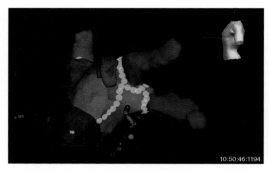

Figure 72.4 NavX image showing left lateral view of left atrial chamber, left atrial appendage, and pulmonary venous geometries in a patient undergoing atrial fibrillation ablation. "Shadows" of His bundle and coronary sinus catheters are shown. Lesion markers have been placed circumferentially around pulmonary vein ostia and extending to the mitral valve annulus. The area of the mitral valve annulus has been "cut out" to show its location.

using multiple electrodes from a catheter can decrease the amount of time necessary to create an accurate geometry. NavX allows for the creation of up to 16 different chamber geometries. Multiple geometry formation is especially useful in atrial fibrillation procedures when the creation of pulmonary vein and atrial anatomies is necessary (Figure 72.4). The "Reassign" feature allows for points collected as part of one geometry to be added to a different chamber. This can be useful when creating left atrial and pulmonary vein geometries to accurately display the location of the pulmonary vein ostia. Several investigators have published their experience using the NavX system for atrial fibrillation ablation procedures [14–19].

Diagnostic Landmarking tool

The Diagnostic Landmarking tool allows for the display of electrophysiological data on a three-dimensional map [20]. As the mapping catheter is maneuvered throughout the cardiac chamber, the three-dimensional location, as well as voltage and timing data of each position is saved. The corresponding voltage or activation timing information can be displayed as a color map. A single set of collected points can be used to display the different map types.

The Local Activation Time (LAT) feature allows for a color-coded isochronal map of activation times for each collected catheter location. A surface ECG or intracardiac electrogram is determined by the user to be reference waveform for activation time mapping. The local activation time is determined by the relative timing of the local electrogram on the mapping catheter, as compared to the electrogram timing on the reference electrogram. Activation times are displayed on the map as colors from white to purple, corresponding to earliest to latest activation. A "buffer" of ten beats or local electrograms is saved for each collected catheter location.

The Diagnostic Landmarking tool also has the capability of displaying the voltage data for each collected catheter location. The corresponding map shows the local electrogram voltage information as a color map from grey to purple, corresponding to low to high voltage (Figure 72.5). This feature can be helpful when mapping substrate-mediated tachycardias, such as ventricular tachycardia in patients with a prior myocardial infarction. The Low-voltage Identification tool allows the user to assign electrogram voltages below a specific amplitude to be displayed with a gray color, thus indicating areas of dense scar. Grey points do not interpolate with adjacent color points.

Complex fractionated electrogram maps

One of the techniques currently being investigated for the ablation of atrial fibrillation involves targeting areas of complex fractionated atrial electrograms. Nadamanee *et al.* published a series of

121 patients undergoing ablation using this approach [21]. At 1-year follow-up, 91% remained free of arrhythmia and symptoms. The NavX system includes an automated program to determine and display electrogram fractionation characteristics. The Complex Fractionated Electrogram (CFE) maps can display a fractionation index based on the intervals between multiple, discrete, local potentials. The fractionation characteristics can be displayed as either the mean or standard deviation of local electrogram intervals. Several authors have published their experience using the automated CFE feature of NavX [22,23].

Integration of CT and MRI images

The NavX system allows for three-dimensional models created from CT or MRI to be incorporated into the system for display with a feature called Digital Image Fusion (DIF) [24]. Three-dimensional images that have been previously created on CT or MRI systems can be loaded or the Verismo software can be used to segment or create three-dimensional images from digital "raw" data from CT or MRI. The currently available system allows for side-by-side integration of CT or MRI images with the created anatomical geometry for the comparison of "real" and "virtual" anatomies (Figure 72.6). Future iterations will allow for registration of CT or MRI images with the created geometry and catheter navigation will be displayed on the anatomically accurate three-dimensional map.

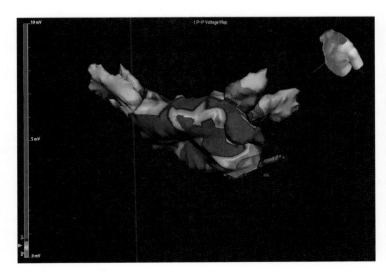

Figure 72.5 NavX Diagnostic landmarking voltage map of left atrium and pulmonary veins in patient with a previous atrial fibrillation ablation undergoing ablation for left atrial flutter. Note possible "gaps" in roofline adjacent to left superior pulmonary vein and near right superior pulmonary vein.

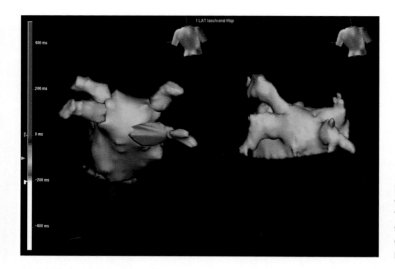

Figure 72.6 Example of DIF technology with NavX system. Three-dimensional CT images are shown side-by-side with NavX geometries of left atrium and pulmonary veins.

Conclusion

The EnSite advanced mapping and catheter navigation system is capable of creation and display of three-dimensional maps displaying anatomically or electrophysiologically based information. The noncontact Array catheter and mapping system allows for single-beat mapping of arrhythmias. The NavX system allows for fast, accurate creation of three-dimensional maps utilizing conventional EP catheters.

References

1. Gornick, C.G., S.W. Adler, B. Pederson, J. Hauck, J. Budd, J. Schweitzer, Validation of a new noncontact catheter system for electroanatomical mapping of left ventricular endocardium. *Circulation*, 1999; **99**: 829–35.
2. Okishige, K., M. Kawabata, S. Umayahara, *et al.*, Radiofrequency catheter ablation of various kinds of arrhythmias guided by virtual electrograms using a noncontact, computerized mapping system. *Circ. J.*, 2003; **67**: 455–60.
3. Higa, S., C. Tai, Y. Lin, *et al.*, Focal atrial tachycardia: new insight from noncontact mapping and catheter ablation. *Circulation*, 2004; **109**: 84–91.
4. Friedman, P.A., S.J. Asirvatham, S. Grice *et al.*, Noncontact mapping to guide ablation of right ventricular outflow tract tachycardia. *J. Am. Coll. Cardiol.*, 2002; **39**: 1808–12.
5. Klemm, H.U., R. Ventura, D. Steven, *et al.*, Catheter ablation of multiple ventricular tachycardias after myocardial infarction guided by combined contact and noncontact mapping. *Circulation*, 2007; **115**: 2697–704.
6. Schumacher, B., W. Jung, T. Lewalter, C.Wolpert, B. Luderitz, *et al.*, Verification of linear lesions using a noncontact multielectrode array catheter versus conventional contact mapping techniques. *J. Cardiovasc. Electrophysiol.*, 1999; **10**: 791–8.
7. Della Bella, P., A. Pappalardo, S. Riva, C. Tondo, Fassini G., Trevisi N., *et al.*, Non-contact mapping to guide catheter ablation of untolerated ventricular tachycardia. *Eur. Heart J.*, 2002; **23**: 742–52.
8. Kaltman, J.R., J.R. Schultz, T.S. Wieand, R.E. Tanel, V.L. Vetter, M.J. Shah, Mapping the critical diastolic pathway in intra-atrial reentrant tachycardia using an automated voltage mapping program. *J. Cardiovasc. Electrophysiol.*, 2006; **17**: 786–8.
9. Krum D., A. Goel, J. Hauck, *et al.*, Catheter location, tracking, catheter chamber geometry creation, and ablation using cutaneous patches. *J. Interv. Card. Electrophysiol.*, 2005; **12**: 17–22.
10. Ruiz-Granell, R., S. Morell-Cabedo, A. Ferrero-DeLoma, R. Garcia-Civera, Atrioventricular node ablation and permanent ventricular pacemaker implantation without fluoroscopy: use of an electroanatomic navigation system. *J. Cardiovasc. Electrophysiol.*, 2005; **16**: 793–5.
11. Earley, M.J., R. Showkathali, M. Alzetani, *et al.*, Radiofrequency ablation of rrhythmias guided by nonfluoroscopic catheter location: a prospective randomized trial. *Eur. Heart J.*, 2006; **27**: 1223–9.
12. Tuzcu, V., A nonfluoroscopic approach for electrophysiology and catheter ablation procedure using a three-dimensional navigation system. *PACE*, 2007; **30**: 519–25.
13. Papagiannis, J., A. Tsoutsinos, G. Kirvassilis, *et al.*, Nonfluroscopic catheter navigation for radiofrequency catheter ablation of supraventricular tachycardia in children. *PACE*, 2006; **29**: 971–8.
14. Rotter, M., Y. Takahashi, P. Sanders, *et al.*, Reduction of fluoroscopy exposure and procedure during ablation of atrial fibrillation using a novel anatomical navigation system. *Eur. Heart J.*, 2005; **26**: 1415–21.

15. Novak, P.G., P.G. Guerra, B. Thibault, L. Macle, Utility of a nonfluroscopic navigation system for pulmonary vein isolation. *J. Cardiovasc. Electrophysiol.*, 2004; **15**: 967.

16. Tondo, C., M. Mantica, G. Russo, *et al.*, A new nonfluoroscopic navigation system to guide pulmonary vein isolation. *PACE*, 2005; **28**: S102–5.

17. Takahashi, Y., M. Rotter, P. Sanders, *et al.*, Left atrial linear ablation to modify the substrate of atrial fibrillation using a nonfluoroscopic imaging system. *PACE*, 2005; **28**: S90–3.

18. Estner, H.L., I. Deisenhofer, A. Luik, *et al.*, Electrical isolation of pulmonary veins in patients with atrial fibrillation: reduction of fluoroscopy exposure and procedure duration by the use of a non-fluoroscopic navigation system (NavX*). *Europace*, 2006; **8**: 583–7.

19. Sherzer, A.I., D.Y. Feigenblum, S. Kulkarni, *et al.*, Continuous nonfluroscopic localization of the esophagus during radiofrequency catheter ablation of atrial fibrillation. *J. Cardiovasc. Electrophysiol.*, 2007; **18**: 157–60.

20. Mangrum, J.M., J.P. Hummel, J. Temple, *et al.*, Initial experience with contact-mapping using the Ensite diagnostic landmarking tool. *Heart Rhythm*, 2005; **2**: S317.

21. Nademanee, K., J. McKenzie, E. Kosar, *et al.*, A new approach for catheter ablation of atrial fibrillation: Mapping of the electrophysiologic substrate. *J. Am. Coll. Cardiol.*, 2004; **43**: 2044–53.

22. Verma, A., P. Novak, L. Macle, *et al.*, A multicenter prospective study of ablating complex fractionated electrograms (CFEs) during atrial fibrillation (AF) using a novel automated mapping algorithm: acute effects on AF and efficacy as an adjuvant strategy. *Heart Rhythm*, 2007; **4**: S348.

23. Wu, J., I. Deisenhofer, A. Luik, *et al.*, Automatic 3D mapping of complex fractionated atrial electrograms (CFAE) in patients with paroxysmal and persistent atrial fibrillation. *Heart Rhythm*, 2007; **4**: S347.

24. Piedad, B.T., J.R. Bullinga, J.S. Sethi, D.S. Holmes, N.E. Bernstein, L.A. Chinitz, *et al.*, Cardiac CT imaging used in conjunction with a non-fluoroscopic navigation system (NavX) for atrial fibrillation ablation. *Heart Rhythm*, 2005; **2**: S172–3.

CARTO XP: tips and tricks

William (Marty) Castell, BS, RCIS

CARTO XP: mapping tips for AV nodal reentrant tachycardia

- Create an anatomical map of the right atrium. Activation mapping is not required.
- Display both proximal and distal bipolar intracardiac electrograms on CARTO XP Annotation Viewer window. Display of both M1–2 and M3–4 bipolar electrograms will assist in bracketing the His bundle.
- Place the catheter in the His bundle position. Confirm His bundle location by visualization of intracardiac electrograms.
- Acquire and apply Point Tags to 5–10 His bundle anatomically located points.
- Continue deflecting the catheter downwards identifying the most inferior His bundle location.
- Define the coronary sinus ostium (CS OS). Locate the anterior, posterior, superior, and inferior aspect of the CS OS.
- Consider applying a vessel tag of the coronary sinus. It may be helpful to visualize the location of the vessel on the anatomical map.
- Rotate the catheter anteriorly. Define the tricuspid valve annulus (TVA) at anatomically different locations (e.g., 3, 6, 9, and 12 o'clock).
- Using a left anterior oblique (LAO) projection in the Map Viewer screen, visual intersection of the CS OS point tags and His bundle point tags can be used to identify the slow pathway region.

Electroanatomical Mapping, 1st edition. Edited by A. Al-Ahmad, D. Callans, H. Hsia and A. Natale. © 2008 Blackwell Publishing, ISBN: 9781405157025.

- A right lateral view in the Additional View screen will be helpful in determining catheter tip orientation in relationship to the CS OS.

CARTO XP: mapping tips for focal right atrial tachycardia

- In sustained right atrial tachycardia (AT), acquire and apply Point Tags to the anatomical landmarks (i.e., superior vena cava [SVC], inferior vena cava [IVC], TVA, CS OS, and His bundle).
- Apply Point Tags to other areas of interest (e.g., RA appendage, crista terminalis, double potentials, and fractionated electrograms).
- Begin acquiring points at the SVC–RA junction followed by point acquisition down the lateral RA wall to the IVC using a sweep and drag catheter motion.
- Repeat this technique of point acquisition by moving the catheter from the SVC down the septal, posterior, and anterior walls for accurate chamber reconstruction.
- Consider the Hot and Cold mapping approach (i.e., low-density chamber sampling in the right atrium to identify global intracardiac electrical activation). Concentrate mapping in the region of early activation to localize the focal site of origin.
- RA chamber map reconstruction: approximately 50–100 points. Activation sampling of all chamber regions and landmark areas are necessary.
- Once the region of early activation is identified, consider decreasing the Fill Threshold to 10 mm, allowing for high-density mapping of the focal area.
- Annotation Viewer window setup: display at least two body surface electrograms, bipolar M1–2 and

M3–4, unipolar M1, and a stable and reproducible intracardiac reference (e.g., coronary sinus).
• If the tachycardia has varying cycle lengths, alternative mapping strategies must be considered.
• If the tachycardia has a change in morphology, beginning a new map must be considered.
• Consider high-output pacing of the distal catheter electrodes to observe diaphragmatic movement and phrenic nerve stimulation.

Note:
• A highly diffuse area of red coloring (early activation) on the right atrial septum may be suggestive of a left-sided tachycardia.
• Point acquisition in the coronary sinus may be useful in determining a right versus a left-sided origin.
• Point acquisition in the left pulmonary artery may also helpful to localize a focal AT originating from the left pulmonary veins.
• If early-meets-late areas are detected on the map (colored dark red and overriding color interpolation), consider reentry versus focal in origin.

CARTO XP: mapping tips for isthmus-dependent right atrial flutter

• Activation mapping for accurate three-dimensional chamber representation.
• Use LAO view in Map Viewer screen to visualize medial/lateral catheter tip position.
• Use right anterior oblique (RAO) or right lateral view in Additional View screen to visualize anterior/posterior catheter tip position.
• Begin acquiring activation points at the SVC–RA junction followed by point acquisition down the RA lateral wall to the IVC using a sweep and drag catheter technique as described earlier.
• Repeat the point collection process by moving the catheter from the SVC down the septal, posterior, and anterior walls.
• Focus point collection in the anterior RA chamber.
• Acquire TVA points at the 1, 3, 6, 7, 9, and 12 o'clock positions.
• Apply Point Tags on the IVC identifying the most anterior and posterior aspects of this structure.

• Apply Point Tags identifying anatomical landmarks such as the His, CS OS, double potentials, and fractionated atrial electrograms.
• Consider applying a Vessel Tag of the coronary sinus to the map for easy landmark identification.
• RA chamber map reconstruction: approximately 50–100 points recommended.
• Once the RA map is complete, rotate the map in the Map Viewer screen to a LAO caudal projection. In the Additional View screen, rotate the map to an RAO or RL projection.

CARTO XP: mapping tips for accessory pathways

• Configure the mapping system annotation setup specific to the approach or protocol used (i.e., atrial pacing mapping the ventricular insertion site; ventricular pacing mapping the atrial insertion site; induce and map the tachycardia; or, map in Sinus Rhythm for earliest intracardiac ventricular activation.
• Decrease the Fill Threshold to 6–8 mm.
• Display in the Annotation Viewer screen bipolar M1–2, M3–4, and unipolar M1.
• Recommend placing the catheter in the desired chamber and applying Point Tags identifying the His bundle location.
• Map the entire annular ring for accessory pathway bracketing and localization.
• High-density map (6–12 points) in the area of early activation.

CARTO XP: mapping tips for right ventricular outflow tract ventricular tachycardia (RVOT)

• Activation mapping during sustained ventricular tachycardia.
• Advance the catheter into the right ventricle and begin point acquisition using the sweep and drag technique making sure to sample and reconstruct the entire chamber.
• Point acquisition of tachycardia beats only (catheter manipulation may provoke mechanically produced beats, i.e., ventricular premature contraction).
• Apply Point tags to all anatomical landmarks (i.e., pulmonic valve, tricuspid valve, and His bundle).

- Right ventricular chamber map reconstruction: approximately 50–100 points recommended.
- If hemodynamic intolerance during tachycardia, consider the Hot and Cold mapping approach (i.e., low-density chamber mapping to identify global intracardiac electrical activation). Concentrate mapping in the region of early activation to localize the focal site of origin.

Note:
- A highly diffuse area of red coloring (early activation) on the right ventricular septum may be suggestive of a left-sided tachycardia.

CARTO XP: mapping tips for ischemic related monomorphic left ventricular tachycardia

- Strategize the mapping approach (i.e., Voltage mapping in sinus rhythm or Activation mapping during monomorphic ventricular tachycardia or a combination of both maps).
- In sustained hemodynamic tolerant monomorphic left ventricular tachycardia, create an Activation map with point acquisition and chamber reconstruction using the sweep and drag catheter technique. Sample the entire left ventricular chamber creating a high-density activation map.

- Consider a system setup using predetermined multiple maps to add and collect data, that is Sinus Rhythm Voltage Map; Activation Map(s) one for each VT induced having different cycle lengths.
- Apply Point Tags labeling all anatomical landmarks (i.e., mitral valve annulus, His bundle, scar, anterior and posterior Purkinje potentials, double potentials, fractionated electrograms, and aortic cusp/LV outflow location.
- LV chamber reconstruction: 200–400 points recommended.
- If mapping during sinus rhythm, create a scar-related bipolar voltage map which displays the peak-to-peak voltage value (mV) at each acquired point. These points are then color coded (low voltage = red; high voltage = purple).
- Maximum and minimum voltage criteria as defined by EP lab criteria (e.g., minimum bipolar voltage = 0.5 mV; maximum bipolar voltage = 1.5 mV).
- Pace-mapping during sinus rhythm: label all sites with identifying information (i.e., 10/12) body surface ECG match. Paced sites resulting in noncapture, despite high output, should be labeled with Point Tags as Location Only or Scar.
- Recommend an RAO projection in the Map Viewer window and an LAO projection in the Additional View window.

Index

265